The Autoimmune Brain

The Autoimmune Brain

A Five-Step Plan for Treating Chronic Pain, Depression, Anxiety, Fatigue, and Attention Disorders

DAVID S. YOUNGER, MD, DrPH, MPH, MS

ROWMAN & LITTLEFIELD
Lanham • Boulder • New York • London

This book represents reference material only. It is not intended as a medical manual, and the data presented here are meant to assist the reader in making informed choices regarding wellness. This book is not a replacement for treatment(s) that the reader's personal physician may have suggested. If the reader believes he or she is experiencing a medical issue, professional medical help is recommended. Mention of particular products, companies, or authorities in this book does not entail endorsement by the publisher or author.

Published by Rowman & Littlefield
An imprint of The Rowman & Littlefield Publishing Group, Inc.
4501 Forbes Boulevard, Suite 200, Lanham, Maryland 20706
www.rowman.com

6 Tinworth Street, London SE11 5AL, United Kingdom

British Library Cataloguing in Publication Information Available

Library of Congress Control Number: 2019949770

ISBN 978-1-5381-1770-5 (cloth : alk. paper)
ISBN 978-1-5381-6629-1 (pbk. : alk. paper)
ISBN 978-1-5381-1771-2 (electronic)

∞™ The paper used in this publication meets the minimum requirements of American National Standard for Information Sciences—Permanence of Paper for Printed Library Materials, ANSI/NISO Z39.48-1992.

Contents

Preface

Pain and suffering, commonly thought of as the consequence of personal injury, connotes the physical and emotional impact of a severe or incapacitating neurological illness. How neurological illness can be prevented, as well as the way you recognize it and live with it or fight back, are major themes of *The Autoimmune Brain*. In short, I start with the premise that illness is a departure from health and wellness. Further, that the effects of infectious microbial invasion, the commonest trigger of illness, elicits a prominent immune response influenced by one's genetics and early infant or adolescent allergies, mold exposure, and metabolic insults. While post-infectious immunity has been known for quite some time, only recently has it been simplified to *I*-Cubed (*I*nfection -> *I*mmunity -> *I*nflammation). Add to this the concept of epigenetics, where environmental insults modify the way cells use DNA instructions, and we have a recipe for concern. When detrimental genes are unsilenced in the DNA of cells, there is a risk for present and future illness. However, passed on to future generations, the same scenario accounts for affliction of future generations, such as when a physically or mentally ill parent gives rise to similarly stricken offspring. However, the buck can stop here when you take control over brain and immune health through a simple five-step process: *T*est, *A*pply, *P*articipate, *E*at smart and exercise, and *S*urvey yourself, home, and environment (abbreviated TAPES).

My insights into the origin, diagnosis, treatment, and prevention of neurological illness stem from my formative training and practice as a clinician in neurology first at Columbia University and then New York University's School of Medicine and Public Health. I added two new accolades by joining the staff of the City University of New York Sophie Davis School of Medicine in the Department of Neuroscience, and the doctoral program in Health Policy and Management. As I recognized that my insights could benefit countless others, this book took form in numerous conversations with colleagues and close friends. I hope that it benefits a generation of parents, families, and caregivers, and especially children, whose resilience never ceases to amaze and inspire me.

My agent Carol Mann, and executive acquisition editor Suzanne Staszak-Silva, have all been supportive of this book from its inception to production. Pam Liflander showed me how to transform my writing style into a more inviting prose. However, it would not have been possible without the support of my wife, Holly, and my sons Adam and Seth, who indirectly participated in every phase of its creation, as truly a work in progress over the past two years, by allowing me the time and inspiration I needed to research and write it.

David S. Younger MD MPH MS
August 4, 2019

Preface to the
Paperback Edition

When I first wrote *The Autoimmune Brain*, my goal was to introduce readers to the complexities of illnesses that, on the surface, seemed to be neurological or neuropsychiatric in nature, but in many cases stemmed from a triad of triggers: infection, poor immunity, and inflammation. I refer to this as I-Cubed (I^3), which describes the downstream multiplier effect that is the basis for post-infectious autoimmunity and the cause of many brain-based symptoms. Readers then learned how to apply my 5-step TAPES protocol to take charge of their health and reverse disease by testing for autoimmunity, applying appropriate immune modulation and pain therapy, participating in therapies to alleviate stress and improve your mental health, eating smart and exercising, and surveying your home and environment for toxins.

While thousands of individuals have since benefited from these insights, no one could have predicted that *The Autoimmune Brain* would be such a timely asset during the COVID-19 pandemic. My research, along with that of others in the field, has found that I-cubed offers a realistic explanation of how infection-triggered neuro-inflammatory disturbances of the immune system result from the body's response to this virus and the resulting cytokine storm.

This paperback edition of *The Autoimmune Brain* now includes a detailed explanation of the phenomena known as Long COVID and Long Haulers. It explains why people who were infected with COVID often continue to exhibit symptoms such as PTSD, depression, anxiety, insomnia, OCD, chronic pain, chronic fatigue, POTS, and neurocognitive disorders for months after they were first infected. What's more, I explain that while its consequences may be ascribed to the immune response to the virus, it is important to recognize the psychological stresses associated with this pandemic that can also lead to symptoms. With these new additions, my hope is that Long Haulers, along with the countless others who are affected by I-cubed, will be able to find the relief they are looking for.

David S Younger, MD, DrPH, MPH, MS
October 2021

Abbreviations

AA	Alcoholics Anonymous
Aβ	amyloid beta
ACE2	angiotensin-converting enzyme 2
ACh	acetylcholine
ACT	Acceptance and Commitment Therapy
AD	Alzheimer's disease
AE	autoimmune encephalitis
ALA	aminolevulinic acid
ANS	autonomic nervous system
ASD	autism spectrum disorder
ASO	anti-streptolysin
ATP	adenosine triphosphate
BBB	blood-brain barrier
B-cell	bone marrow derived cell
BID	twice daily
BP	blood pressure
CAH	congenital adrenal hyperplasia
CBD	cannabidiol
CBT	cognitive behavioral therapy
CD	Celiac disease
CDC	Centers for Disease Control and Prevention
CFS	chronic fatigue syndrome

CIDP	chronic inflammatory demyelinating polyneuropathy
CNS	central nervous system
COVID-19	2019-coronavirus-2-pandemic
CRH	corticotrophin releasing hormone
CSF	cerebrospinal fluid
CT	computed tomography
CVID	common variable immune deficiency
CYP21	21-hydroxylase gene
DBT	dialectical behavioral therapy
DHA	docosahexaenoic acid
DNA	deoxyribonucleic acid
EDS	Ehler-Danlos syndrome(s)
EEG	electroencephalogram
EMG	electromyography
ENF	epidermal nerve fiber
ENS	enteric nervous sytem
EPA	eicosapentaenoic acid
°F	degrees Fahrenheit
FODMAP	fermentable oligo-, di-, mono-saccharides and polyols
GABA	gamma aminobutyric acid
GABHS	group A beta-hemolytic streptococcus
GAD65	glutamic acid decarboxylase 65
GFD	gluten-free diet
GI	gastrointestinal
HBV	hepatitis B virus
HCV	hepatitis C virus
HLA	human leukocyte antigen gene
HE	Hashimoto's encephalopathy
HMBS	hydroxymethylbilane synthase gene
HPA axis	hypothalamus-pituitary-adrenal axis
HR	heart rate
HT	Hashimoto's thyroiditis
5-HT	5-hydroxytryptamine
IAg	intraneuronal antigen
IBD	inflammatory bowel disease
ICD 10	tenth edition of the International Classification of Diseases

I-Cubed	I^3 (Infection -> Immunity -> Inflammation)
IgA	immune globulin A
IgG	immune globulin G
IgM	immune globulin M
IL	interleukin
IQ	intelligence quotient
IVIg	intravenous immune globulin
Kg	kilograms
LE	limbic encephalitis
LNB	Lyme neuroborreliosis
MDD	major depressive disorder
ME	myalgic encephalomyelitis
MHC	major histocompatibility complex
microRNA	microribonucleic acid
Mg	milligrams
MMR	measles, mumps, and rubella
MIS-C	multisystem inflammatory syndrome
MRI	magnetic resonance imaging
mTBI	mild (concussive) traumatic brain injury
MS	multiple sclerosis
MU	million units
NAA	N-acetylaspartate
NCS	nerve conduction studies
NE	norepinephrine
NMDA	N-methyl-D-aspartate
NSAID	nonsteroidal anti-inflammatory drug
OCD	obsessive-compulsive disorder
OH	orthostatic hypotension
PANDAS	pediatric autoimmune neuropsychiatric disorders associated with streptococcal infections
PANS	pediatric autoimmune neuropsychiatric syndrome
PASC	post-acute sequelae of SARS-COV-2
PCR	polymerase chain reaction
PD	Parkinson's disease
PET	positron emission tomography
PNS	peripheral nervous system

POTS	postural orthostatic tachycardia syndrome
PTLDS	post-treatment Lyme disease syndrome
PTSD	post-traumatic stress disorder
PUFA	polyunsaturated fatty acids
Q4H	every 4 hours
Q8H	every 8 hours
ReA	reactive arthritis
RNA	ribonucleic acid
SAg	surface antigen
SARS	severe acute respiratory syndrome
SARS-COV-2	SARS-coronavirus-2
SBP	systolic blood pressure
SCIg	subcutaneous immune globulin
SEID	systemic exertion intolerance disease
SFN	small fiber neuropathy
SNRI	selective serotonin-norepinephrine reuptake Inhibitor
SpA	spondyloarthropathy
SPECT	single photon emission computed tomography
SSRI	selective serotonin reuptake inhibitor
TAPES	Test, Apply, Participate, Eat, Exercise and Survey
T-cell	thymus derived cell
THC	tetrahydrocannabinol
TID	three times daily
T1D	type 1 diabetes
T2D	type 2 diabetes
TM	transcendental meditation
TNF	tumor necrosis factor
TNXB	tenascin X gene
VGKC	voltage gated potassium channel

Introduction

There are millions of people who experience issues related to brain health—depression, attention issues, anxiety, forgetfulness, fatigue, and even chronic pain—yet can't figure out what's causing their problems and can't find any relief. They may have seen a myriad of physicians, many of whom do not take their complaints seriously, or worse, turn to the easy, albeit inappropriate fix of antidepressants or antianxiety medications. Traditional medications, supplements, or other therapies haven't worked. No matter what their age—from children to teens to seniors—these people and their loved ones are frustrated, scared, and confused by their continued poor health.

Countless others display more severe psychiatric symptoms that seem to come out of nowhere: obsessive-compulsive behaviors, suicidal thoughts, tics, and mood swings reminiscent of bipolar disorder. Sometimes, the person affected is the only one that notices a change to the way they think or feel, and they suffer in silence. Alternatively, they reach out to try to get help and are all too frequently misdiagnosed.

I know this scenario all too well. As a neurologist, I see a wide variety of illness and injury, and one common thread is that all of my patients suffer from changes to their cognition, mood, memory, chronic pain, and the ability to balance or sleep. Most of my patients have already seen a primary care physician who has tried to relieve their symptoms or complaints, but has come up short. Often, they've been to well-reputed medical institutions like Johns

Hopkins, Columbia, or Weil Cornell. They may have seen an infectious disease specialist, a rheumatologist, a psychiatrist, or psychologist. Each of these specialists is well intentioned, but they cannot get to the root of the problem. The reason is that few physicians outside of neurology realize the deep connection between autoimmunity and brain health.

In fact, very few neurologists connect common brain health symptoms to the changes in the immune system caused by bacterial, viral, and parasitic infections. Yet the cutting edge of medicine is finding that recurrent bacterial infections initiated during childhood, or dormant viruses that become reactivated, are common culprits. Parasites, ranging from Lyme, Babesia, or even *Entamoeba histolytica* and pinworm (ingested from eating unwashed salad or raw fish) can also cause brain health symptoms.

I also know that people who have undiagnosed autoimmune diseases including celiac, lupus, chemical and drug sensitivities, food allergies and sensitivities, and environmental exposures to mold often have brain health symptoms that can include depression, fatigue, brain fog, and psychological distress. In fact, a change in personality, behavior, coping style, and one's emotional state may be the first clue that there is a health problem brewing somewhere else in the body. I'm here to tell you that, together, we can explore these connections and end the hopelessness many patients feel that they'll never be understood or cured.

This book is the culmination of more than a decade of research. It will explore many questions with the intention of creating a clear link between these two phenomena and discover for each of us which is the active instigator. In other words, do the consequences of an autoimmune insult cause brain symptoms, or are such symptoms pieces of the puzzle that characterize the nature of the insult?

Equally important is the understanding of stress and how it affects health. Everyday stress can affect the most basic molecules of the body, contributing to the inflammatory response integrated by immunity. Traumatic stress (whether physical or emotional) is just as important as infections and genetics, and together they may be tangled factors important in initiating autoimmune disease and the resulting brain health symptoms. This revolutionary idea is the basis behind my theory, I-Cubed. This book is meant to walk you through the trifecta of infection, immunity, and inflammation, and show how all three may be affecting your health.

A LITTLE BIT ABOUT ME

My interest in brain health began when I was a teenager, and the interest continued through my medical training. I worked as a counselor at a summer camp before I went off to college. It was a very special place: a camp dedicated for kids that at the time were unfortunately labeled as retarded. I saw that in many cases, these kids had both mental and physical health issues, yet back in the 1970s, no one really knew what caused the retardation.

I went to college at the University of Michigan, and I was so passionate about working with such children that I planned to major in education. Later on, I decided to become a physician. My specialized training focused on neuromuscular diseases, which I pursued during my first fellowship. I did a second fellowship in electroencephalogram testing and epilepsy, where I got a chance to monitor premature infants and childhood epilepsy. Then I did another fellowship in clinical trials and started on a master's degree in public health: I felt that it wasn't enough just to take care of single individuals—I believe that physicians should be part of the larger healthcare policy conversation. I am board certified in Internal Medicine, Neurology and Public Health, with postdoctoral training in public health and epidemiology.

Along the way I published many clinical papers, primarily focusing on neuroimmunology—the intersection of neurology and how the immune system affects the nervous system. I was among the first to bring to the nation's awareness the triad of infection, immunity, and inflammation, abbreviated as "I-Cubed," and known more commonly by physicians as *post-infectious autoimmunity*.

The concept of I-Cubed emerged following the explosion in the number of people with autoimmune diseases or similar conditions, especially those associated with Lyme disease. I put together a Lyme disease research program to investigate the mechanism of Lyme and its relationship to a poorly developed Lyme vaccine. We knew at the time that the Lyme vaccine stimulates immunity but it doesn't cause infection. However, the vaccine had to be taken off the market because patients were developing complex neurological syndromes. During the program, we realized that the damage was caused by inflammation during a post-infectious autoimmunity-like mechanism. The synthetic constituent that was meant to stimulate an immune response to protect a person against Lyme was actually causing a stronger reaction, affecting the brain and nervous system.

I then took this hypothesis to the next step: it seemed logical to me that this same response happens in most autoimmune diseases. In fact, now we know that I-Cubed is a very common mechanism for body protection, and it's also a legitimate mechanism for a prolonged autoimmune response.

Since then I have become even more intrigued by the early onset of mental illness in adolescents, especially in relation to infectious illness. My current research focuses on the genetic basis of predisposition for autoimmune conditions related to mold or food allergies/sensitivities, bacterial and viral exposures people may have had apart from infection, or people that are at risk for celiac disease or other neurogenetic family influences, and how the brain is affected. Sadly, I continue to see that most practicing physicians are not putting these two issues together, and they are viewing brain health issues as solely psychological or psychiatric problems. But to my mind, these are medical cases that need to be medically treated.

Early and accurate diagnosis is most important for our littlest patients. Children are set up for failure unless they're properly diagnosed. For instance, a delay in proper treatment means that children are missing school, or they're being given an accommodation instead of a diagnosis so they don't flunk out, but there's very little movement forward on addressing the cause and providing proper treatment. With the rising incidence rates of depression and anxiety disorder among kids worldwide, and with children missing an average of two weeks or more of school for experiencing "bad days," it's time to look for new causes.

The patients I'm seeing now are already in crisis, as I've become the physician of last resort, who can finally solve the problem because of my diversity in training. I pride myself on being that physician who will continue probing until we find answers. This means tirelessly addressing each of my patient's symptoms and looking at each person from a whole-body standpoint.

But identifying the cause of a problem is only the first step. Many sufferers are misdiagnosed with an autoimmune or chronic disease because the symptoms are often the same, but the testing and treatment are vastly different. While most physicians still believe that a virus will only last 24 to 48 hours so don't worry about administering antibiotics, they are doing their patients a grave disservice. To reverse these diseases and restore overall health, I have developed cutting edge treatment protocols centered on immune modulatory therapy with gammaglobulin (known as IVIg) that have been adopted by physicians across the country. This unique treatment plan has become the most widely employed immune-modulating agent for autoimmune neurological disorders. Even though IVIg has been around for a long time, most physicians were not generally applying this to infectious processes. They apply it to pure autoimmune disorders like connective tissue diseases or the rheumatologic realm. Yet I have seen firsthand that gammaglobulin has the benefit of being a generally efficient way of enhancing the whole immune system in a more holistic healthy way.

HOW THIS BOOK WORKS

The good news is that it's never too late to understand the underlying mechanism that's keeping you feeling crazy, out of control, forgetful, and exhausted. This book is written for the millions of sufferers, their families, and their physicians: for anyone experiencing changes to their cognition, mood, or sleep patterns. If you've tried everything and you're still not quite right, take this book to your physician. Teach him or her about I-Cubed, and get the right treatment that will put you or your family member back on the path to health.

The core of this book is identifying what your symptoms are and then determining if you are suffering from an autoimmune issue that is causing brain health problems. My protocol will give you a new approach toward investigating your problem, understanding the mechanisms for your illness, point you toward appropriate further testing to confirm your suspicions, and ultimately give you the therapeutic tools to restore health and reverse disease. Some treatment options require medical supervision; others do not.

This new paradigm for identifying illness and resetting the immune system can be summarized by the acronym *TAPES*:

- *Test* for the most likely autoimmune disturbance right at home, and discover how a specific autoimmune response may be affecting brain health.
- *Apply* immune-modulating therapies (under a physician's care) that will address both the immune response and changes to brain health.
- *Participate* in the most effective behavioral/therapeutic options to reduce stress and reverse fatigue, anxiety, depression, and memory loss.
- *Eat and Exercise* to restore brain health, alleviate pain, and enhance the immune system.
- *Survey* your home for chemical exposures and remove mold, heavy metals, and other allergens that can stand in the way of a full recovery.

LET'S GET STARTED

The next chapter breaks I-Cubed into its separate parts so that you can understand the relationship between the parts of the triad: infection, immunity, and inflammation.

I

UNDERSTANDING I-CUBED

1

The Basics of Brain Health and Autoimmunity

A neurologist focuses on three core areas of health:

- The central nervous system (CNS): the brain and the spinal cord
- The peripheral nervous system (PNS): the network of nerves leaving the brain and spinal cord, continuing to the muscles and the skin
- The autonomic nervous system (ANS): how the brain and body regulate functions beyond our conscious control, such as temperature, digestion and metabolism, breathing, and heartbeat.

Everything we do, all day long (and at night as well) involves these three systems either independently or in an overlapping fashion. It takes a very careful coordination of these three basic systems in order to maintain focus, balance, and high cognitive function. Picture in your mind the classic image of a Native American riding a horse, with bow and arrow drawn, tracking his prey across the desert plains. When our bodies are used at their fullest potential, we are coordinating intellect, balance, and muscular coordination.

You can categorize your physical symptoms into one of these three systems. The ANS has three branches: the sympathetic nervous system, the parasympathetic nervous system, and the enteric nervous system. The sympathetic nervous system controls hormonal output and the "fight or flight" response, whereas the parasympathetic nervous system monitors our ability to "rest and digest." The ANS, also known as the visceral organ nervous system, is connected with motor functions, causing muscles to contract or relax; and balances circulatory function throughout the body, including the brain, through its control of blood vessels, which is referred to as *vascular tone*. ANS disorders can disturb normal bladder, bowel, and sexual function and lead to deficient vital signs with postural changes. Other common manifestations include temperature dysregulation, skin color changes, hair loss, increased or decreased perspiration, and as you'll see later in this chapter, postural orthostatic tachycardia syndrome (POTS) and orthostatic hypotension. The third branch of the ANS, the enteric nervous system, operates autonomously yet communicates with the CNS by using brain chemicals called *neurotransmitters*, most of which are identical to the ones found in the CNS.

CNS disorders are typically uncommon and degenerative, and have very specific features that will facilitate a correct diagnosis. Amyotrophic lateral sclerosis, better known as Lou Gehrig disease, is a CNS disease that unmistakably involves the brain and spinal cord. It is suggested by the symptom cluster of progressive pharyngeal and limb weakness, wasting and twitching, and spasticity that results from degenerative loss of upper and lower motor neurons of the brain and spinal cord.

PNS disorders also have typical features. Guillain-Barre syndrome, abbreviated GBS, causes unmistakable ascending weakness and sensory loss over days resulting in progressive paralysis. More common expressions of PNS disturbance are the numbing and tingling sensations of neuropathy that occur with diabetes or Lyme disease.

Neurological symptoms may be unmistakable for a given disorder; in other circumstances, they may not be so straightforward. For instance, each of these three systems can be affected by, or create, symptoms like fatigue, forgetfulness, cognitive changes, panic attacks, and anxiety. Panic attacks can be thought of as an outflow of the ANS, a sort of unrestrained hyperactive dynamic state that cannot be controlled.

BOX 1.1

THE BRAIN-SKIN CONNECTION

The skin is your largest organ and has both peripheral and autonomic components. The skin has pain and temperature receptors, which belong to the peripheral nervous system and are catalogued as *small fibers* because they can only be seen with a microscope. A second type, small nerve fibers are classified as part of the autonomic nervous and sensory systems. The *small autonomic fibers* are "effectors" in nature, originating in the brain's hypothalamus, descending through the brain stem, spinal cord, and along spinal roots to insert themselves into peripheral nerves of the limbs and trunk where they gain access to skin organs such as sweat glands, blood vessels, and hair follicles. By contrast, *small sensory fibers* in the skin are "receptive" in nature, provide pain and temperature receptors that transmit information to the brain in the opposite direction by connecting with the peripheral nerves and spinal roots, up through the spinal cord and brain stem on their way to the brain for conscious appreciation of these senses.

BRAIN HEALTH BASICS

The brain's anatomical and physiological functions are governed by a highly complex system of connections that enable us to experience our environment and to think deeply. Higher cortical functions, including consciousness and how we process thoughts and actions, occur in the cerebral hemispheres, the largest parts of the brain. These hemispheres are divided into various lobes. The *frontal lobe* occupies most of the brain and is the home for both higher cortical function and executive function (decision-making). Other lobes have existed long before the frontal lobe evolved its higher functionality. These include the temporal lobes, occipital lobe, and parietal lobe, where specialized functions related to memory, vision, and sensation interacts. The brain physically connects to the body at the brain stem, which then continues into the spinal cord. Both the brain stem and the spinal cord are thought of as extensions of the brain, much like a mushroom cap and its stem.

The higher functioning parts of the brain send electrical signals to the rest of the body through the spinal cord and the nerve system, and then the different lobes use sensory information to create thoughts, memories, and language. For example, sensory input from the environment—touch, vision, hearing, taste, smell, and feel—become integrated in the brain. The spinal cord then relays out its information to the limbs via nerve routes, and then along peripheral nerves into the arms and legs, or other organ systems. This is how we can see a fire and know to move away from it quickly.

CNS oversight of ANS mechanisms reside in the hypothalamus, which is an area in the brain that lies just above the brain stem. The CNS relies on the vascular system, through which it releases specialized molecules from the hypothalamus that travel to the pituitary gland, which prompts the release of hormones into the bloodstream. Similar to trains leaving from Grand Central Station to distant destinations via their separate tracks, peripheral autonomic nerve fibers branch throughout the body and influence the function of visceral organs. One such integrated circuit is the hypothalamic-pituitary-adrenal (HPA) axis, which is responsible for the release of the cortisol and two catecholamines: adrenaline, which is important in generating energy during stressful situations, and norepinephrine, which is the main neurotransmission of the ANS that instructs the visceral organs including the heart, lungs, and blood vessels.

UNDERSTANDING BASIC BRAIN CHEMISTRY

Brain cells, or neurons, are located both at the surface and deep into the brain, and they connect to each other in an intricate fashion. Neurons send electric brain commands to all of our muscle functions and are the heart of the CNS. The messaging is accomplished through the transmission of neurotransmitters, which are primarily hormones that are released upon activation. Most neurotransmitters are created in unique parts of the brain, and then widely distributed throughout the nervous system. Their proliferation is a sign of good health, and a lack of neurotransmitters is directly correlated to poor health. For example, the neurotransmitter dopamine is created in the part of the brain known as the *substantia nigra* and is essential for maintaining normal motor tone. When one has low levels of dopamine, he or she can develop diseases like Parkinson's disease, which is a degeneration of muscle tone.

The most common neurotransmitters are serotonin, dopamine, histamine, epinephrine, and norepinephrine, and each is paired with receptor sites in both the brain and the body. In a perfectly working brain, there is a balanced flow of neurotransmitters, but this is not always the case. However, doctors are not really concerned with enhancing neurotransmitter production or suppressing it. Instead, they focus on affecting brain chemistry by making a person's output more efficient, which better facilitates communication within the brain where messages might get lost. For example, antidepressant drugs, like selective serotonin reuptake inhibitors (SSRIs), act upon a specific class of receptors for serotonin, making them more available to receive serotonin. Other drugs, like serotonin–norepinephrine reuptake inhibitors (SNRIs), inhibit the receptors from receiving serotonin and norepinephrine. Most doctors do not differentiate between the SSRIs and SNRIs on the basis of which neurotransmitter uptake they wish to favor when dealing with depression alone. However for neurologists and psychiatrists, the choices are more important.

HOW THE IMMUNE SYSTEM INTERACTS WITH THE BRAIN

A second component of brain health involves the immune system. Your immune system is a delicate and complex network of interacting cells, cell products, and cell-forming tissues that protects the body from foreign invaders. These invaders, known as *antigens,* can be viruses, bacteria, and other foreign bodies (mold, dirt, etc.) that cannot be accepted into the body as normal. Your immune system resides primarily in the gut, the liver, and the bloodstream. It also is found in the brain in the form of glial cells.

Glial cells primarily protect the *blood–brain barrier* (BBB), the passageway and filtration system of the brain. The BBB also acts as a firewall protecting the brain from normal distresses. The barrier is one vascular endothelial cell thick, which is just enough to protect the entire CNS within the skull from intruders but porous enough to permit a healthy interchange of vital molecules that the brain uses as nutrients for its normal metabolism. Yet certain infections head directly toward the brain, including Lyme disease, certain forms of herpes, Whipple disease, and others, regardless of their point of origination.

Each location of the immune system has at least two arms: the cellular, or innate, immune system, which reacts by creating small proteins that affect their surrounding cells known as *cytokines* to destroy a threat; and the humoral, or adaptive, immune system, which is called in as a backup support system. When faced with any antigen, the innate/cellular immune system produces cytokines, which can recognize and then destroy whatever they consider threatening.

If the cellular arms' defensive strategy cannot get the job done, the humoral/adaptive immune system kicks in, launching *antibodies*. These antibodies specifically match the organ where the invader is located. When these antibodies attack an organ in their attempt to attack an invader, and do not stop, an *autoimmune response* has been created.

Because there are so many likely foreign invaders, each time your immune system launches an attack it retains the memory of that event in the major histocompatibility complex (MHC) playbook. The MHC genes, residing on chromosome 6, act as both a playbook and your immune system's dictionary. When your immune system is overwhelmed by a very powerful, or new, invader, that playbook is ever more crucial to guide an appropriate immune response. The result is an inflammatory response: an increased secretion of blood containing immune-enhancing white blood cells and antibodies. The inflammation is directed to an area of the body or brain that requires healing.

Whether, when, and how we will unleash the autoimmune response is determined by our genetics, the microbiome of bacteria in our gut, and our body burden—our ability to respond appropriately to antigens. No two people will react to an infection or other immune system insult in the same way. However, when the innate immune system is worn out, increasingly higher levels of antibodies are released to attack and destroy the antigens, and this process creates excess inflammation as well as collateral damage caused by antibodies attacking both the antigens and the organ they are found in. Slowly and insidiously, that autoimmune response can cause damage and eventually a disease state.

Autoimmune diseases are thought to affect one in five American women and one in seven men. Yet this estimate accounts for only those with a clinically diagnosed autoimmune disease. The truth is that the autoimmune response can affect the brain and nervous system before symptoms that affect the body manifest. And much like high blood pressure, obesity, and other persistent illnesses, autoimmune diseases need to be managed daily with an individualized program that works. Moreover, the only way to lessen an autoimmune reaction is by resetting the immune system and regulating its efforts so that the body's inflammation can reduce. The only way to reduce inflammation and restore proper functioning is by proactively following a low inflammatory plan to reduce the daily buildup of unnecessary inflammation.

The autoimmune response can occur anywhere in the body, and when it comes to the brain, there are two types of autoimmune brain antibodies that can wreak havoc. The first lie on the surface of brain cells, and a second targets the nucleus, or center, of the neuron. Certain symptoms, such as seizures, irritability, and mood disorders, are commonly related to cell surface reactions and reversible functional changes in the mind, whereas those related to intraneuronal damage cause irreversible loss of function, such as memory loss and loss of intellect. The latter are referred to as neurodegenerative due to the progressive nature of the insult, resulting in neuronal death.

Inflammation is a complex biological response fundamental to how the body deals with injury and infection, to the elimination of the initial cause of cell injury and its ultimate repair. Unlike a normally beneficial acute inflammatory response, chronic inflammation leads to tissue damage and ultimately its destruction. It often stems from an inappropriate immune response. Inflammation in the nervous system, so-called neuroinflammation, especially when prolonged, can be particularly injurious. While inflammation per se may not cause disease, it contributes importantly to disease pathogenesis across both the PNS and CNS. The existence of extensive lines of communication between the nervous system and immune system represents a fundamental principle underlying neuroinflammation. Immune cell–derived inflammatory molecules are critical for regulation of host responses to inflammation. Although these mediators can originate from various non-neuronal cells, important sources of divergent neuropathologies appear to be microglia and mast cells, together with brain neurons. Understanding neuroinflammation requires an appreciation of cell–cell interactions as integral parts of the inflammation process. Within this context the mast cell occupies a key niche in orchestrating the inflammatory process, from initiation to prolongation.

Inflammation affects the brain, making the BBB more permeable. When the brain is attacked by the immune system, it creates an inflammatory state recruiting mediator molecules including interleukins (ILs) and complement proteins that irritate and disrupt the BBB; and when this happens, it causes the brain to mount its own immune response. This is a worst-case scenario: not only is it an insult on the barrier, but its substances can go from the bloodstream through the barrier, into the brain and spinal area. Different autoimmune issues affect the brain differently, because specific antibodies dictate a different syndrome and a different brain response. But in general, excess inflammation caused by an autoimmune response can make it difficult for the brain to respond quickly and adequately. There may be explicit instructions on how to execute a complex task that cannot get through because the brain activity has become slower. For instance, the autoimmune disease Hashimoto's encephalopathy (HE), associated with Hashimoto's thyroiditis (HT), is an autoantibody-mediated inflammatory disorder of both the thyroid gland and brain, associated with disruption of the BBB and resulting cognitive and neuropsychiatric symptoms.

There are more than 300 known autoimmune diseases, and any one of them can cause either direct or indirect brain health symptoms. One of the major goals of achieving better brain health is reducing systemic inflammation: just by reducing inflammation, your brain health symptoms may reverse. Later, through the testing chapter, we'll be able to point you toward what diseases you actually might have. Even things as basic as arthritis can lead to profound immune responses in the body. Many cause what's called constitutional symptoms, which is fatigue, lethargy, loss of energy, a thinking disorder, and even depression. The role autoimmune dysfunction plays in some neuropsychiatric illnesses has been investigated as far back as the 1930s, when autoantibodies to the brain were first reported in a schizophrenia patient.[1] Since that time, there have been reports of specific autoimmune responses to antigens in psychosis, affective disorders, and other neurobehavioral abnormalities.[2,3]

Systemic disorders with possible involvement of the nervous system include a variety of diseases with presumed inflammatory and autoimmune mechanisms, including systemic inflammatory disorders with a genetically defined dysregulation of the innate immune system, as well as systemic autoimmune disorders characterized by alterations of the adaptive immunity such as autoantibodies and autoreactive T-cells. Although more commonly diagnosed in adults, all of these diseases can manifest in childhood and some as early as infancy. Neurological involvement may represent the initial manifestation, and nearly every neurological symptom can be caused by a postinfectious inflammatory autoimmune trigger akin to I-Cubed. These include various bacterial infections (strep, mycoplasma, tuberculosis, Lyme disease, syphilis, and *Salmonella*), viral infections (coronaviruses, Epstein-Barr, cytomegalovirus, *Varicella*, parvovirus, enteroviruses, hepatitis B and C virus

(HBV, HCV), West Nile, and human immunodeficiency virus), fungal infections (*Aspergillus, Coccidioides,* and *Toxoplasma*), and protozoal infections. Many systemic diseases such as lupus, sarcoid, scleroderma, inflammatory bowel disease, cancer, and drug and radiation reactions have the capacity to engender immune reactions resulting in inflammatory damage to brain cells.[4]

The HPA axis mentioned earlier is a critical component of the body's response to infection, inflammation, and tissue injury. As you learned, immune reactions typically begin in the CNS in response to stimuli, and immunocompetent cells such as monocytes, lymphocytes, and macrophages secrete a full range of cytokines and other inflammatory mediators to combat the invader. Three specific cytokines, IL-1 and IL-6 and tumor necrosis factor(TNF)-α, are released via the HPA axis. It is becoming clear that inadequate activation and reduced responsiveness by the HPA axis due to an underlying brain disturbance may impact on a person's capacity to withstand infectious invasions or a developing autoimmune disorder.

A change in personality, behavior, coping style, and one's emotional state may be the first clue to abnormalities in immune neuroendocrine regulatory function due to activation of cytokines in the brain. Unrecognized and thus untreated, there can be potentially serious consequences ranging from mental changes to stroke.

BOX 1.2

WHEN IT COMES TO SYMPTOMS, WHICH IS THE CHICKEN, WHICH THE EGG?

Is an autoimmune insult causing the brain symptoms? Or are the brain symptoms really a piece of the insult? This is one of the more persistent questions that bother my patients. For instance, many studies on Lyme disease show that if you look at the neuropsychological profile of a patient with chronic Lyme, there may be a mood disturbance; yet it does not bear resemblance to a major depressive disorder. So-called Lyme encephalopathy presents with subtle neuropsychiatric symptoms that can occur months to

(Continued)

(Box 1.2, continued)

years after initial exposure to the tick, *Borrelia burgdorferi* (abbreviated *B. burgdorferi*). For these patients, brain magnetic resonance images (MRI) are usually normal; however, single photon emission computed tomography (SPECT) has been used for more than two decades to successfully monitor the progress of antibiotic therapy.[5] In one study, it was found that SPECT imaging demonstrated reduced blood flow to the brain, particularly in frontal subcortical and cortical regions where it typically increases with a Lyme infection. However, SPECT cannot be used alone to diagnose Lyme encephalopathy or determine its presence in the setting of an active central nervous system infection. Last year, research employing brain positron emission tomography (PET) showed for the first time, evidence of metabolic brain changes related to immunological activation in patients with post-treatment Lyme disease syndrome (PTLDS), manifested as cognitive changes.[6]

THE ROLE OF STRESS IN AUTOIMMUNITY

Our mental stress changes the way brain chemicals are produced and transmitted. There is a mechanism for unleashing and producing proteins that have a genetic role in conveying information and modifying your gene production of proteins and neurotransmitters.

The hippocampus is the mood and memory area, and also the home of ANS function. Stress modifies the transmission of neurotransmitters by changing the profile of certain microribonucleic acids (microRNAs) in the hippocampus, which has an effect on other parts of the brain. These are the small noncoding RNA molecules that contain roughly 22 nucleotides and function as silencers and regulators of messenger RNA that conveys genetic information from DNA, to specify the amino acid sequence of the protein products of gene expression through the process known as *post-transcription gene regulation*.

One such pathway is the cholinergic anti-inflammatory pathway, which acts as a link between the brain and the immune system in response to immune challenge, and controls the inflammatory response through its interaction with receptors expressed on macrophages. MicroRNAs are necessary for cholinergic anti-inflammatory action by inhibiting the production of pro-inflammatory cytokines. The microRNAs are sitting strategically in the immune system, arbitrating immunity and its effect on the brain.

Mental stress modifies neurotransmission by changing the profile of certain microRNA's in the brain. One particular microRNA, miR-124, is present in a variety of brain disorders[7] such as multiple sclerosis, Parkinson's disease, Alzheimer's disease, amyotrophic lateral sclerosis, and other brain disorders. It has been shown that animals affected by psychological stress and exhibiting symptoms alter their immune response activation associated with upregulation of miR-124. MicroRNAs also have unique expression profiles in cells of the immune systems functioning as "negotiators" between the CNS and immune system.

Traumatic stress can lead to inflammation and cause its own autoimmune response. The inordinate stress or profound stress we feel could be as dangerous to the brain as an infection. Because everyone reacts to stress differently and the way you handle stress is how resilient you are, this book provides ways for you to modulate your stress to become more resilient.

POST-INFECTIOUS AUTOIMMUNITY: I-CUBED

A concept that has risen in importance among immunologists and other physicians intrigued by the role of the immune system has been the recognition that an infection, whether it is a new infection or a chronic infection that is latent in the body, is a primary antigen, which stimulates the immune system. On a molecular level, an infection can undergo constant changes in its genetic composition in response to environmental influences while it is living in the body, and the body has mechanisms for adjusting the response it will have to the infectious organism. What's more, different areas of the nervous system can all be involved when there is a post-infectious autoimmune event, leading to a variety of symptoms, often far from the original site of infection.

Organisms are learning how to invade us more efficiently. In fact, we're not even aware of probably 90 percent of the real complex structure of unique organisms that have yet to be identified. For instance, Whipple disease is a nervous system illness that was found only by testing spinal fluid or in tissue of the intestine, even though it is primarily a nervous system disease.

Stress modifies the triad of infection-immunity-inflammation and can affect the brain with potentially disastrous consequences on cognition and mood. A salient example occurs with a chronic HCV infection.[8] Afflicted patients experience a range of symptoms including depression, fatigue, and neurocognitive deficits. Depression in particular may be reactive to increased psychosocial stress or other physical symptoms of advanced HCV. Patients at an early stage of HCV infection report more depressive symptoms and fatigue than the general population. Similarly, specific neurocognitive deficits occur in early stage HCV infection and are independent of the presence of depression or encephalopathy.

Changes to the brain's structure associated with HCV may explain these symptoms. These changes may arise from infiltration of the brain, penetrating the BBB, by peripherally induced cytokines, as well as direct neuropathic effects of HCV particles. These particles can create an inflammatory response, alter neurotransmitter levels, disrupt hormonal output, and release neurotoxic substances. Any and all of these may subsequently lead to abnormal neuronal conduction and function in areas of the brain governing affective responses, emotional processing, motivation, attention, and concentration. Although medication will treat the HCV virus, they will not reverse symptoms of depression, fatigue, and neurocognitive deficits.

Meet Sandy

Sometimes, patients can have issues in all three brain systems, and that problem can stem from autoimmunity. My patient Sandy was 17 when he first came to see me, and he had already suffered from numerous concussions from playing basketball. He had been out of school for six months and only had enough energy to lie on his bed for most of the day. Sandy's mom was convinced that his lethargy was either caused by a concussive head injury or that he had a serious psychological problem.

When Sandy came into my office, I immediately saw an overweight young man who had memory and mood issues and was exhibiting neuropsychiatric problems, suggestive of CNS involvement. However, it was unclear whether he was traumatically brain injured. He complained of tingling, numbness, and limb weakness, a sure sign of PNS involvement.

I decided to do a full autoimmune blood panel, and we discovered that Sandy had a number of immunologic issues, including HT, and antibodies to the brain, referred to as an HE. He also had numerous ANS-related blood flow defects we could see on brain SPECT, meaning that there was damage to the BBB caused by a yet unknown autoimmune inflammatory process.

These results led me to think that something outside of the brain was affecting the nervous system, which would have crossed the brain through the BBB. The concussion might have exacerbated the problem, but was not the cause. We later postulated that HT leading to HE was damaging the hippocampus, the seat of mood and memory.[9] The concussion must have opened up the BBB, so what would otherwise have remained a silent disease he would have lived with forever without knowing it became the target of our therapy. Ultrasound-guided biopsy of the thyroid showed HT, and PET/MRI showed hippocampal hypometabolism with focal changes suggesting inflammation.

We treated the autoimmune brain changes with intravenous immuno-globulin therapy, known as an IVIg protocol, which is featured throughout this book, and I prescribed corticosteroids (prednisone) to lower the inflammation connected to HE, and supplemental thyroid medication to address the HT directly. Today Sandy was off the sofa and back at school after IVIg therapy. Treating the HT and HE, and lowering his inflammation with both prednisone and IVIg helped him to lose weight and increase his energy level. Once the pathways from the brain via the HPA axis were addressed, his metabolism was readjusted, he was able to achieve a stabilization of all his vital signs, and the dizziness went away. Sandy graduated high school, and he's preparing for college, but he's got enduring psychological issues that are kept in check with antidepressants and behavioral therapeutic care. It's going to take some time before he's back to feeling good all the time, but he is well on his way.

POSTURAL ORTHOSTATIC TACHYCARDIA SYNDROME

One increasingly recognized ANS disorder is postural orthostatic tachycardia syndrome (POTS), which is a perfect example of how I-Cubed affects your health. It is also associated with other conditions including joint hypermobility, chronic fatigue, neuropsychiatric disturbances, painful small fiber neuropathy, and altered nervous system immunity.

POTS is an ANS disorder because it involves poor vascular tone, which limits the ability of the blood vessels in the legs to move blood upward toward the heart and head against gravity, which is what happens when you suddenly stand upright from a lying or sitting position. The symptoms of POTS are due to the abrupt and sustained rise in heart rate when moving from sitting to standing.[10] These patients typically have peripheral neuropathy that could contribute to autonomic impairment. Their successful management depends upon carefully considering all of the possible underling metabolic, infectious, genetic, and autoimmune triggers.

POTS causes seemingly cardiac symptoms such as rapid palpitations, light-headedness, chest discomfort, and shortness of breath, as well as non-cardiac symptoms including brain fog, headache, nausea, tremulousness, generalized weakness, and blurred or tunnel vision.[11] Many patients with POTS are diagnosed with migraine headaches, as well as mottling of the legs from the feet to above the knees.[12] People with POTS also complain of non-specific gastrointestinal symptoms of abdominal pain, nausea, and irritable bowel syndrome, and urinary complaints including bladder symptoms.[13] More generalized complaints in patients with POTS include exercise intolerance and sleep disturbance. Patients frequently report that their symptom onset following acute stressors including pregnancy, traumatic event, surgery, or a viral illness.

However, this does not mean that POTS is stress-induced. Instead, I believe that it is an underlying biological dysfunction that manifests during stressful situations. The difference is that people with POTS are not suffering from an emotional disorder; they are suffering from a hard to diagnose medical event. In fact, it is not uncommon for my patients with POTS to tell me that when they were youngsters, they suffered from fear of public speaking because they regularly experienced the sensation of their heart pounding in their throat.

I've also found that POTS can occur with other autoimmune disorders, which is no surprise—you'll learn that many people with an autoimmune disorder will experience others throughout their lifetime. Patients with POTS have a higher prevalence of unexplained chronic fatigue,[14] as well as a heightened prevalence of joint hypermobility disorders.[15,16]

Meet Rue

Rue was a 19-year-old freshman at college on a basketball scholarship. Her father is a pastor and she has 11 siblings. Yet the normal stresses of a life balancing her family, college studies, and a team sport were compounded when her older brother and his wife died of drug abuse. Their only child was being raised by Rue's father, and Rue developed such a strong bond with her that she referred to the 2-year-old as "my daughter."

Rue came to see me when her teammates commented that she was unable to pick up her feet, which was when she finally admitted to herself that she felt constantly winded and had heart palpitations just rising from the bench. This was followed by burning and stinging sensations in the feet. After a few more weeks, she noted pain in the arms and hands.

When she came to see me, Rue told me that during the time her niece started living with her family, she had a bout of mononucleosis followed by walking pneumonia, both of which were unrecognized and treated erroneously as asthma. She also commented that she hadn't been getting along with her college roommate and had recently moved out of the dorm. All of these stress factors (infection, family turmoil, and college life) preceded the onset of her physical complaints. She did not consider herself depressed but admitted to thoughts of self-harm.

I noticed that Rue also had mottling of the skin, impaired pain and temperature sensation in her feet, absent reflexes, and was turning one foot inward as she walked, which clearly was affecting her balance. I performed a tilt table test to confirm that she had POTS. This type of test is the best way to reproduce the characteristic features of POTS. During the test, Rue experienced anxiety, palpitations, fatigue, weakness, and burning, which confirmed the diagnosis.

I started Rue on a low dose of a long-acting beta-blocker, metoprolol (Toprol XL), to control her POTS, and I encouraged her to increase her fluids and dietary salt to increase intravascular blood volume. Appointments were made for her to undergo electrodiagnostic studies, epidermal nerve fiber studies, and further screening for metabolic, autoimmune, genetic and infectious triggers that may have contributed to her declining health. The trigger of her POTS, presumptive painful small fiber neuropathy, awkwardness of gait with turning of one foot, and the visible aspect of her incapacity to play basketball were undoubtedly related to the earlier infectious exposures, compounded by recurrent stressors, making this a form of post-traumatic stress disorder. After I explained these causative factors, she felt relief in knowing that she might soon improve. However, she continued to progress to bilateral foot drop that required braces. It turned out that the neuropathy was still progressing as indicated by electrodiagnotic studies and epidermal nerve fiber (ENF) analysis of a punch biopsy of skin along the calf and thigh. I am watching her carefully and monitoring her progress on weekly IVIg therapy, physical therapy, and an antidepressant utilizing an SNRI combined with psychological counseling.

2

How the Brain Develops

Parents often come to my office concerned that even the smallest changes to their child's brain health will spiral into severe cognitive changes. The truth is, brain development can be altered by physical sickness, and different regions of the brain can be affected in both the short and long term. By identifying which illnesses can affect brain function, and the likely signs to look for, we can control damage before it creates long-term problems. Therefore, we need to do everything we can while the brain is still developing and has a lot of *plasticity*, or ability to change, in order to address brain insults.

The key to early identification is to listen carefully to what your children— or your own body—is trying to tell you. When teens are feeling crazy, confused, and tired, you need to make sure their voice is heard. Often, children and adults don't have the language to express the changes they experience in their thoughts and feelings. When this happens, they become *involutional*, looking inwards for answers instead of expressing frustrations or concerns. Or they turn away from conventional medicine and use the internet for answers. When these avenues are exhausted, often without finding relief for symptoms, patients and parents alike can become increasingly frustrated, confused, and create feelings of abandonment. In the worst cases—particularly for teens— they reach the point of despair and may act out suicidal thoughts.

Unfortunately, I see many patients in their teen years that are depressed, suicidal, or practice self-harm behaviors, like cutting. A perfect example was a teenage girl who had unrelenting depression throughout junior high and high school. The parents were at a complete loss, and when they finally came to see me, the daughter had dropped out of college her freshman year and cut herself on every limb. Testing confirmed that she had Lyme disease, which we know has severe neurologic components. Once she started on the proper treatments, her mental health challenges slowly subsided. The hopelessness went away, and we were able to deal with the immune challenges that came up from the Lyme disease, as well as her psychiatric illness and thought disorder.

With suicidal teens on the rise, it prompts the question: is there a growing trend of anxiety and disillusionment, or is the trend an increase in undetected yet reversible illness? If these teens have been misdiagnosed, are we just coming to it too late, and therefore only observing the final stages, which might be suicide or suicidal ideation? In this book, you will learn exactly how infections trigger inflammation, which is often a precursor to mental illnesses that could be prevented.

I believe that in many cases, the I-Cubed triad of infection, immunity, and inflammation is the underlying cause of a complex problem that is reaching near-epidemic levels. Parents can play a big role in prevention by bringing their children to the attention of neurologists and psychiatrists. The next question is when did these changes in the brain systems first occur?

THE PRIMACY OF INFANCY
The concept that brain development relates to cognitive development first came to my awareness during a freshman introductory neuroscience course at Columbia College of Physicians and Surgeons in 1978 when Nobel Prize Laureate Professor Eric Kandel started the class saying, "behavior depends on the formation of appropriate interconnections among neurons in the brain." He would go on to write the bible of neuroscience.[1,2] That astute statement foreshadowed for me the enormity of human neuroscience research that blossomed during the period from 1990 to 2000, which we now refer to as the Decade of the Brain. This era led to a variety of activities, publications, and programs aimed at introducing politicians, educators, private and public funding agencies, and the general public to cutting-edge applied neuroscience research.

One revelation that attracted attention was the process of *cortical synapto-genesis*—how different functions of the brain connect to each other and create neural circuitry. This process starts during gestation and continues shortly after birth. Throughout this time, the developing brain can be influenced by the mother's health, especially regarding problems that can occur with infections. This is especially true during the first trimester. We now know that infections like the Zika virus can cause a brain insult to a fetus that can lead to a slowing of brain development, physical deformation, and possibly fetal death. Other viruses that pregnant women can be exposed to such as mumps and measles can be equally damaging, possibly leading to childhood emotional problems or other subtle neurological issues.

Over the past two decades, the field of developmental neuroscience has discovered meaningful links between specific brain processes and cognitive developments. With a relatively complete wiring diagram for several important regions of the brain, researchers and cognitive neuroscientists have laid the foundations for important cognitive capabilities that sequentially emerge in infancy. Each well-defined period of exuberant synaptogenesis marks the emergence of a specific new cognitive capacity. Moreover, with each new refinement in the morphology of the brain, during so-called *critical periods*, a new function is achieved. All of these maturational processes occur concurrently throughout all cortical regions of the brain throughout motor, sensory, language, and visual lobe cortices, tapering by the age of 7 years. We now know that a healthy newborn baby has more synaptic connections than at any other point in life. If he or she makes it through a full-term pregnancy healthy, they are born with a brain that has twice the amount of neurons and synapses it needs to function. Over the next several months and years the infant goes through a critical period of neural pruning, which strengthens the most used neuronal connections until the brain approximates that of an adult. During this time, the developing brain is so plastic, or changeable, that most adverse insults—whether infectious or physical—can be overcome.

There is a popular notion that in the period of birth to age 3, when brain circuits are being formed, parents have a unique opportunity to build better brains and offset mental illness,[3] in what has become the battle cry of early childhood experts to proclaim "use it or lose it." In reality, brain power has little, if anything, to do with the wealth of early childhood experiences most parents strike to provide.[4] The movement to embrace 0 to 3 years has nonetheless focused our attention on infants and toddlers basic needs for safety, nourishment, nurturing and loving attachments, and to strive as a society to expand maternity leave and provide childcare for working parents, and prekindergarten for all 3-year-olds. Parents should feel comforted in knowing that the new brain science holds the promise of curing, or at the least, ameliorating the most challenging early childhood I-Cubed disorders by harnessing the nervous system's innate plasticity and regenerative capacity.

Expert pediatricians note that breast milk has evolved to provide the best nutrition, immune protection, and regulation of growth, development, and metabolism for the human infant. Breast milk is critical in compensating for developmental delays in immune function, and it is responsible for reducing the permeability of the intestine. The favorable gut microbiome, which appears to be a function of the interaction between human milk's microbiota, is endowed with important antimicrobial activity. Healthy infant microbiome promotes integrity of the intestinal barrier and competitively inhibits pathogen binding, preventing inflammatory responses that can later result in neurological complaints.

Autoimmunity can affect brain development in utero. In 2017, researcher Michael Nash and his colleagues[5] described that the bacteria found in a developing infant's gut, which we refer to as the *microbiome*, affects not only their metabolism, but the maturation of the gastrointestinal tract, immune system function, and brain development. Initial seeding of the neonatal microbiota occurs through maternal and environmental contact. Maternal diet, antibiotic use, and cesarean section can all affect the offspring's microbiota composition, at least temporarily. The mother's nutrient intake was found to regulate initial perinatal microbial colonization, a paradigm known as the "Restaurant" hypothesis. This hypothesis proposes that early nutritional stresses alter both the initial colonizing bacteria and the development of signaling pathways controlled by microbial mediators. These stresses fine-tune the immune system and metabolic homeostasis in early life, potentially setting the stage for long-term metabolic and immune health.

Dysbiosis, an imbalance or a maladaptation in the microbiota, can be caused by several factors, including dietary alterations and antibiotics. Dysbiosis can alter biological processes in the gut and in tissues and organs throughout the body. Dysregulated development and activity of the immune systems, driven by early dysbiosis, could have long-lasting consequences such as an increased risk of developing autoimmunity, affecting both the brain and the body.

BRAIN DEVELOPMENT THROUGH THE TEEN YEARS

The human brain undergoes further profound changes during the first two decades of life. Key developmental events, such as the initial growth of axons during the second trimester in utero or the pruning of excess synapses during childhood and adolescence, are critical in sculpting the anatomical wiring.[6] These developmental changes in neuronal connectivity parallel the maturation of social, cognitive, and motor skills that begin at birth and continue through young adulthood.[7] Any changes to the process of normal development increase the risk of neurodevelopmental disorders such as autism spectrum disorder, attention-deficit hyperactivity disorder, and schizophrenia.[8]

The complete network of neuronal connections comprising the human brain is called the *connectome*.[9] Connections within this intricate network are distributed unevenly, such that certain network elements possess a relatively large number of connections, marking them as putative network *hubs*.[10] Brain hubs facilitate the integration of functionally specialized and anatomically disparate neural systems, in a role supported by their tendency to form long-range connections,[11] and their position within the brain, which suggests that they mediate a large fraction of signal traffic.

BRAIN DEVELOPMENT AS AN ADULT

The brain never stops changing or growing, even into adulthood and throughout the lifespan. Researchers refer to this continuous increase in neuronal development as *neurogenesis*, and it is the promise of some of the most exciting findings in medicine today. The formation of new neurons in the adult central nervous system has been recognized as one of the major findings in neuroanatomical research. One particular area of the brain that holds promise for continued neurodevelopment and eradication of disease is the hippocampal formation.[12] Many cellular features from this region emphasize that hippocampal neurogenesis suffers changes with normal aging and, among regulatory factors, physical exercise and chronic stress provoke opposite effects on cell proliferation, maturation, and survival. Considering the numerous functions attributable to the hippocampus, increasing or decreasing the integration of new neurons in the delicate neuronal network might be significant for reversing declines in cognition and treating mood disorders, especially depression.

Your current health doesn't have to be your destiny. By following the TAPES program outlined in part II of this book, you can literally increase your neuronal development and repair your brain. At the same time, you will be lowering inflammation and addressing your immune system to bring it into balance, possibly for the first time in your life.

Meet Thomas

Thomas was a 16-year-old boy who had life-long joint hyperextensibility: he was double jointed. By the time he was 12, he already had several bouts of strep throat, and a year later was diagnosed with Lyme disease. About that time he began to manifest anxiety. He started whispering instead of speaking loudly, and a year later experienced *selective mutism*, where he would only speak at home. He stopped eating to the point that when he came to see me, he had lost 30 pounds, and his muscles were so weak that he was dragging his right foot. The MRI we ordered showed that his brain was normal, but his throat tonsils were critically enlarged. I advised a tonsillectomy and started him on intravenous immunoglobulin therapy. Electrodiagnostic studies of his legs and left arm showed peripheral sensory neuropathy. Blood tests showed that he was at risk for Celiac disease, but not Lyme.

Thomas's health improved with aggressive holistic management of all the possible contributors to his brain disturbances, including strep infections, gluten exposure, and commencing intravenous immunoglobulin therapy to keep his immune system modulated and pediatric autoimmune neuropsychiatric disorder associated with group A beta-hemolytic streptococcus infection (PANDAS) in check. Along with his physical health, these treatments also address his cognition and mood. His anxiety has lessened, and he no longer speaks in whispers.

3

Is My Problem Neurological or Psychiatric?

The fields of neurology and psychiatry, both of which explore and treat the brain, have been artificially separated by the divergence in philosophical approaches, research, and treatment methods. A psychiatrist focuses on the narrow area of mood disorders, and the medications and therapies that can address them, and they may not take into account the range of neurological insults that can translate into a psychological/psychiatric problem. Personality disorders, depression, and other mood disorders are some of the issues a psychiatrist is more likely to address, especially if these are the only symptoms that present. A neurologist has to be an expert in the mechanical workings of the brain systems as well as an expert in all matters dealing with psychiatry. In short, a neurologist has to recognize when a patient has a psychiatric problem with a neurologic basis, or neurologic problem leading to psychiatric manifestations.

However, the two fields are increasingly converging, creating a third one, which we call *neuropsychiatry*. We refer to psychological symptoms as neuropsychiatric when they occur in the setting of a neurological disorder. This clarification recognizes that some brain health symptoms are likely caused by brain dysfunction, and failing to recognize that overlap may be at the detriment of making a solvable diagnosis. For instance, as soon as a psychiatric patient presents with symptoms of a neurological disorder, such as limbic encephalitis, which has memory disturbances as a symptom, then the diagnosis is transformed from strictly psychiatric or neurologic to neuropsychiatric. It stands to reason that a precipitous onset of psychiatric symptoms should always prompt the search for a simultaneous medical process, such as underlying infectious or autoimmune disorder.

Yet how many individuals are dismissed by physicians doubtful that vague complaints of pain, fatigue, anxiety, and sleep problems are not authentic and instead represent attention seeking behavior? Faced with a patient who presents with unexplained and disproportionate pain, Patterson and Grelsamer[1] point out that physicians are tempted to diagnose a low pain threshold, malingering, poor coping, anxiety, or other emotional condition. However, there are a variety of bona fide conditions that should be ruled out before prescribing watchful waiting. Any of these symptoms may be the first sign of a neuropsychiatric or mental illness, loosely defined as a condition that significantly affects a person's cognition, behavior, perception, and emotions. Once present, they impact how the affected person interacts with other people. Undiagnosed and therefore untreated, it quickly worsens over time, leading to serious and debilitating social and work impairments as evidenced by increased days sick at home and out of work.[2]

In my experience, many physicians, even those with the best of intentions, lump fatigue, anxiety, and sleep difficulty along with weight loss, fevers, sweating disturbance, chronic pain, fatigue, and malaise as "constitutional" in nature, even though each of these may be the first sign of a neuropsychiatric process.

Growing research points to the overlap between psychosis and neuropathological processes associated with immunological dysregulation as well as inflammation.[3] A 2018 discovery of antibodies against synaptic and neuronal cell membrane proteins, such as the N-methyl-D-aspartate (NMDA) receptor antibody, points to the etiological connection between autoimmunity and subsequent risk of depression and psychosis. In this way, autoimmunity may masquerade as drug-resistant primary neuropsychiatric disease, depending upon the anatomical area and intrinsic connections affected, as well as the nature and severity of the immunological insult.

Epidemiological studies have also shown a strong bidirectional relationship between autoimmune disorders and psychosis,[4] meaning that the two can occur together. One 2017 study from the same research group showed a positive correlation between brain-reactive antibodies associated with autoimmune disorders and the subsequent development of psychosis.[5]

In this chapter, we will parse through these different areas of neurology to help you identify the underlying cause of your concern. In the most recent mental health surveillance among US children from the past decade compiled by the Centers for Disease Control and Prevention, derived from two national surveys (the National Health Interview Survey and the National Health and Nutrition Examination Survey) and the National Center for Health Statistics, mental illness of all types, from bipolar depression to psychosis to autistic spectrum disorders, was on the rise.[6]

We now know that 20 percent of children aged 12 to 17 years are at risk for developing a mental health disorder.[7] A review of recent research[8] shows that irrespective of the cause, 18 percent of children experience at least ten days each year that can be categorized as "sad days," and 28 percent of high school children report feeling so sad or hopeless every day for two weeks or more that they stopped their usual activities. These "bad days in school" may be a clue to either an underlying physical illness or a diagnosable mental illness. They might indicate a brain chemical imbalance with a genetic, infectious, or autoimmune component.

Scientists say that the roots and spectrum of mental illness are present earlier than suspected in children. Once mental illness develops, it can become a regular part of a child's behavior and more difficult to treat.

BRAIN STRUCTURE AFFECTS MOOD

A number of brain regions appear central to understanding how we develop mood disorders. Anatomical, neurophysiological, functional neuroimaging, and neuropsychological evidence[9] have shown that certain anterior limbic and related structures, including the orbitofrontal cortex and amygdala, are involved in emotion, reward valuation, and reward-related decision-making but not memory. In this emotional limbic system, there are visual, olfactory, and auditory stimuli networks, and other reinforcements of emotion derived from taste, touch, and pain. Complementary evidence indicates that the hippocampus system receives information from neocortical areas about spatial location and objects, and can rapidly associate this information together by the different computational principles of automatic association to inscribe memory but not emotion.

More specifically, the hippocampus is one region that has recently received significant attention in mood disorders research.[10] It is involved in learning and in the consolidation of discrete short-term memories to their cortical storage for the long term. It is considered to be highly plastic, or malleable, and sensitive to stress.

Hippocampal neurons encode receptors to all of the major neurotransmitters or brain chemicals, including gamma-aminobutyric acid (GABA), acetylcholine (ACh), norepinephrine (NE), and serotonin. Antidepressant medications work by directly addressing increased or decreased production of these brain chemicals, as well as creating new neuronal connections through the process of neurogenesis. Animal studies also suggest that antidepressant medications may in fact protect hippocampal integrity.

A compelling source of data that shows the importance of hippocampal integrity in thwarting mental illness has come from MRI studies of the brain of individuals with depression[11] and autoimmune encephalitis (AE).[12] In 2017, I hypothesized that depressed patients and those with progressive AE have significantly decreased hippocampal volumes compared with age-matched controls. A small hippocampus in comparison to whole brain volume suggests early disturbed neurodevelopment or the effects of a neurotrophic illness such as infection or autoimmunity. The notion that a small hippocampus confers vulnerability to stress-associated disorders and mental illness is suggested in twin studies that support the role of genetic factors.[13] Mechanisms by which genetic vulnerability are expressed leading to a small hippocampus are not well understood.

Meet Maisy

The case of my patient, Maisy, drives home the point that psychiatric disorders can be associated with brain dysfunction and altered immunity. Maisy thought she was going crazy because seemingly out of nowhere she developed vertigo, headaches, and a full-blown psychotic break at age 21 that was accompanied with auditory and visual hallucinations. She had already seen a psychiatrist who identified that she had bipolar disease and prescribed psychotropic medication.

Maisy also went to see a holistic physician who identified possible Lyme exposure. She was prescribed antibiotics, yet continued to have pain and numbness in her face, hands, and feet, with a relapse of neurocognitive dysfunction. The Lyme medications seemed to contribute to her hallucinations.

Her symptoms were so bad that her doctor admitted her to a hospital that specialized in psychiatric care associated with obsessive-compulsive disorder (OCD), post-traumatic stress disorder (PTSD), and probable bipolar disease. While her therapy included a hodgepodge of antidepressants, antipsychotic medications, and cognitive behavioral therapy designed to help her cope with her emotions, every time she went off her antipsychotics, she developed auditory hallucinations.

My neurological examination and spinal tap showed that the Lyme disease was not affecting her health as much as the medications were. However, a new scan employing the radiotracer [18]fluoro-deoxyglucose and positron emission tomography (PET) fused with MRI (PET/MRI) showed mild hypometabolism in the brain hippocampi, areas of the cortex associated with mood and memory disturbances. Once her psychiatric treatment was more closely aligned with the underlying brain dysfunction, she was eventually able to get her life back on track.

AUTOIMMUNITY AFFECTS MOOD

The role of the immune system in the cause of neuropsychiatric illness has been convincingly shown in AE, defined as an autoimmune inflammatory disturbance of vital areas of the brain that is associated with mood and memory. This disease process is localized in the limbic lobe, which includes the hippocampus as the major structure. The past decade has witnessed the emergence of serum autoantibodies directed against antigens present on the surface of limbic system neurons and synaptic-enriched regions of the hippocampus; collectively they can lead to the emergence of neuropsychiatric symptoms. Further supportive of an autoimmune role for the development of AE is the occurrence of novel (meaning new to everyone) serum antibodies that share the property of strong immunolabeling of areas of dense dendritic network and synaptic-enriched regions in the neuropil of hippocampus, sparing most neuronal cell bodies. Not surprisingly, the clinical expression of these antibodies leads to dominant behavioral and psychiatric symptoms and seizures. Newly available brain imaging employing PET/MRI localizes the resultant neuropathology to the hippocampus and medial temporal lobe of the brain in neural circuits believed to be responsible for mood, memory, and neuropsychiatric illness.

A less serious but nonetheless important neuropsychiatric problem is generalized anxiety disorder (GAD). A recent cross-sectional study of about 2,000 community-dwelling people aged 65 or older noted a prevalence of anxiety was 11 percent, with a quarter of individuals reporting their first episode after age 50. While most cases of symptomatic anxiety in the elderly are recurrent, only about a third receive appropriate medical attention. Women are more likely to suffer from GAD, and those that do also experience cognitive impairment, reduced body mass index, low affective support in childhood, psychotropic medication use, major depression, and phobias. It appears that anxiety in later life does not represent the continuing chronic course of early onset illness but has a clinical presentation distinct from generalized anxiety disorder in younger populations with age-specific predictors such as metabolic disorders and chronic diseases including adiposity, respiratory disorders, arrhythmia, heart failure, and cognitive impairment making it a real neuropsychiatric illness.

Although anxiety disorders can be triggered by stressful life and adverse life events, an important and overlooked factor in all age groups, not just the elderly, is dysfunction of the adrenergic and noradrenergic stress systems that comprise the autonomic nervous system. The mechanism of heightened anxiety is purportedly related to a baseline increase in outflow of activity along the hypothalamic-pituitary-adrenal (HPA) axis that leads to the secretion of cortisol and adrenaline into the bloodstream following stressful events. Other patients may have evidence of neuroendocrine dysfunction and overt brain injury.

On the far end of the spectrum are suicidal behaviors and non-suicidal self-injury, both of which are associated with deficits in emotion regulation abilities. Self-injurious behavior may become an attractive option when individuals are unable to identify and utilize strategies that lessen unbearable anxiety or distress. The desire to "feel something, even if it was pain" is a commonly reported motivation for engaging in these behaviors. Anhedonia, a symptom of depression and defined as the inability to feel and experience pleasure and other emotions, appears to link depressive symptoms to self-injurious behaviors. Beyond its status as a core symptom of major depressive disorder, anhedonia is associated with feelings of numbness and emptiness. A growing body of evidence has established a link between anhedonia and suicidality. No doubt there are some individuals who exhibit suicidal and non-suicidal self-injurious behaviors, the treatment of which may be influenced by recognizing infectious and autoimmune risk factors in the emergence of their disease.

FIBROMYALGIA: AN OVERLAP OF NEUROLOGICAL AND PSYCHIATRIC ASPECTS

Fibromyalgia demonstrates the overlap of neurological and psychiatric aspects that can occur within one disease. Fibromyalgia is a chronic, multiple symptom disorder that affects an estimated 2 percent of the population, and it may be linked to viral infections or physical injury. Sufferers experience widespread pain often caused by something that doesn't normally cause pain, such as a light pressure, migratory pain (pain that moves from one part of the body to another), and overwhelming fatigue. And while fibromyalgia has a lot of symptoms in common with other autoimmune diseases, it is not classified as such.

The roots of fibromyalgia can be traced to the early part of the twentieth century with references to "fibrositis," "muscular rheumatism," and "lumbago," terms used interchangeably to describe pain in lumbar spine muscles. During World War II, physicians diagnosed fibrositis in more than three-quarters of soldiers attending military hospitals, often with similar non-specific complaints and symptomatology. Doctors recognized that there were specific painful trigger points, such as along the neck, shoulder, elbow, wrist, palms, low back, and at times in a more generalized distribution. Therapy included non-steroidal anti-inflammatory medications, immobilization of the affected areas, infiltration of trigger points with procaine and corticosteroids, local heat, massage, and postural exercises.

Secondary to pain were the emotional aspects of the disorder, which include unrefreshing sleep, cognitive difficulties, and altered mood. Although the tenth edition of the International Classification of Diseases (ICD-10) lists fibromyalgia as a diagnosable disease and states that it should be classified as a functional somatic syndrome rather than a mental disorder, we know now that some patients with fibromyalgia can have altered immunity and, consequently, brain health symptoms. This is particularly true with those who demonstrate markers of inflammation, notably an elevated erythrocyte sedimentation rate, C-reactive protein, antinuclear antibody, and rheumatoid factor. These people are often diagnosed as having *inflammatory* fibromyalgia.[14]

TESTING OFFERS THE MOST ACCURATE DIAGNOSES

The medical testing outlined in chapter 5 offers some of the best ways that you can determine once and for all if your symptoms are psychiatric or neuropsychiatric in nature. For instance, a compelling source of data has come from MRI of the brain. We can now easily diagnose an AE from newly available brain imaging, including MRI and PET scans. Blood tests that reveal autoantibodies can also be used diagnostically.

Then, with the right diagnosis, treatments can be much more effective. The goal of all such therapies is to enhance neurogenesis and create better synaptic connections. So while it may be a very positive experience to work with a psychotherapist, if your symptoms are biological in nature, you are not medically addressing the underlying cause of your symptoms.

4

Own Your Genetics

Many people who come to see me don't realize that mental health issues have a biological basis. Many of my patients who believe they are depressed, or have been diagnosed as depressed, believe that their affliction is literally all in their head: that they are responsible for feeling the way they do, or that the circumstances of their lives are the cause. However, while that may be the case for a certain subset of people, depression and other mood disorders are real medical issues that have a biological component. What's more, we are living in an age that for the first time in the history of medicine and psychiatry, there is now a wealth of research that has clarified the role of biology in development of mental illness at all stages of life, from childhood to adulthood. We have already touched on the roles that infections and the autoimmune response play, and in this chapter, we will explore the genetics of brain health and how genetics influences infections, inflammation, and immunity.

UNDERSTANDING GENETICS

Our deoxyribonucleic acid (DNA) works like a manufacturing code for the production of all body proteins, giving precise directions for the production and assembly of protein molecules in all body tissues including the nervous system to build our genetic infrastructure. This includes the core of our immune elements in all regions of the body serving both defensive and offensive surveillance roles at "point of entry" for intruders such as in the gut and BBB.

Epigenetics refers to the ability to regulate or modify the underlying DNA sequence by external environmental factors without altering the DNA code itself. In a sense it is the turning on and silencing of risk genes. A good example is multiple sclerosis.[1] Myelin is a lipid-rich structure that protects nerves to avoid leakage of electric signals and to ensure steady electrical impulses along axons. Understanding how the myelination process is programmed, coordinated, and maintained is crucial for developing therapeutic strategies for remyelination in the nervous system. Epigenetic mechanisms have been recognized as a fundamental contributor in this process. In recent years, histone modification, DNA modification, adenosine triphosphate (ATP)–dependent chromatin remodeling, and non-coding RNA modulation are very active areas of investigation. Conceptual frameworks that integrate crucial epigenetic mechanisms with the regulation of oligodendrocyte and Schwann cell lineage progression during development and myelin degeneration in pathological conditions are necessary to treat these debilitating disorders that involve demyelination, such as multiple sclerosis in the central nervous system and neuropathies in the parasympathetic nervous system.

Our genes can also carry mutations, or errors, that can lead to serious illness, especially when it concerns the nervous system. Genetic testing, which will be covered in detail in the next chapter, is the best way to determine if you are carrying specific genes or genetic mutations that are connected to illnesses that affect brain health. Once you determine your risk factor, you can make more informed decisions about your health. For example, knowing that you have a compatible genotype for Celiac disease or depression, with their health implications for the gut, brain, and psyche, should compel you to seek the best defense through dietary gluten restriction and a brain health program to modify your risk.

GENETICS AND I-CUBED

The latest research in molecular genetics explains its influence on the triad of infection, inflammation, and immunity. The body's immune system is encoded in our DNA on chromosome 6 to distinguish itself from infectious foreign invaders. This is integral to the success of the immune response because an immune response unleashed upon the host, perceived as foreign, would cause immense damage. This highly specialized immune function is carried out on successively more complex levels beginning with an innate immune response encoded by human leukocyte antigens (HLA) that recognize microbial peptides within infected cells, tagging them for immediate attack and engulfment by specific killer T-cells and antibodies. An even more sophisticated set of genes encode immune responses to microbial antigens present outside of the cell and elicit the proliferation of T- and B-cell clones, and complement activation that permanently seeks out foreign invaders in carefully orchestrated surveillance missions.

All of the genes involved in our protective immunity have been under immense selective pressure in the past century due to the appearance of new epidemics, such as Zika virus and Ebola virus infection, and the emergence of potentially dangerous resistant strains of common bacterial, viral, and parasitic organisms due to indiscriminate use of antibiotics and multiple drug resistances. HLA genes, which encode our immune system via cell-surface proteins on chromosome 6, have an unusually high rate of variation compared to other genes in the genome, which indicates that we have evolved to combat infectious microbes, and when deficient, genetics may be the leading factor in losing the battle to infections.

Genetic diseases are determined by the combination of genes for a particular trait that are on the chromosomes received from the father and the mother. Dominant genetic disorders occur when only a single copy of an abnormal gene is necessary for the appearance of the disease. The abnormal gene can be inherited from either parent, or can be the result of a new mutation (gene change) in the affected individual. The risk of passing the abnormal gene from affected parent to offspring is 50 percent for each pregnancy regardless of the sex of the resulting child. Because of our unique genetic makeup, each individual can respond differently to particular infections. For example, in the case of Celiac disease, it's possible for just two out of three children in a family, each descended from the same parents that carry the Celiac disease HLA risk alleles, to develop gluten sensitivity.

The loss of tolerance to self-antigens is the starting point for autoimmune diseases which characteristically begin at a relatively young age. There may be either (or both) a genetic predisposition and a preceding viral infection of one of a dozen types (including coronaviruses, herpes, cytomegalovirus, Coxsackie, West Nile, or Zika) that sets it off. One good example is autoimmune thyroid disease.[2] It occurs due to loss of tolerance to thyroid autoantigens thyroid peroxidase, thyroglobulin, and thyroid stimulating hormone receptor, which leads to the infiltration of the gland. T-cells in chronic autoimmune thyroiditis and genetically programmed cell death in thyroid follicular cells cause destruction of the gland. The presence of thyroid peroxidase antibodies is common in Hashimoto's thyroiditis (HT) and Graves' disease (GD), whereas thyroglobulin has been reported as an independent predictor of thyroid malignancy. Cytokine proteins play an important role in autoimmunity by stimulating B- and T-cells, which enhance the inflammatory response.

BOX 4.1

WHEN GENETICS DEFINE INFECTION

The discovery of the bacteria causing Whipple disease, a mysterious infection of the gastrointestinal tract, was a turning point in showing the power of genetics in neurological diagnosis. Classic Whipple disease occurs from an infection with the bacterium *Tropheryma (T.) whipplii*. Whipple disease causes a systemic infection, which unrecognized and untreated most often involves the gastrointestinal tract, heart, and/or brain. Studies showed[3] the location of *T. whippelii* RNA to be most prevalent near the tips of the intestinal villi between adjacent cells, and not intracellular, indicating that the bacillus grew outside cells. However, the organism can also be found in the cerebrospinal fluid in 10 percent to 40 percent of cases who present with neurological or psychiatric symptoms but without gastrointestinal symptoms.[4] When first identified as the causative agent of a neurological disorder almost 25 years ago,[5] it was unclear whether the bacteria *T. whippelii* was a rare member of a normal human microbiome or whether it is introduced to the body through another disease.

THE GENETICS OF THE GUT–BRAIN CONNECTION

Doctors and researchers used to believe that we each have our own genetic code, and it wasn't changeable. You were born, you were dealt this hand, and if your mother had cancer, you were going to have cancer. And if your mother had depression, you were going to have depression. But now we know that epigenetics plays a key role, and that lifestyle influences the way your genes turn on and off. So while you may be predisposed to certain neurological disorders, your lifestyle is going to modulate whether you're going to be affected by them.

One of these lifestyle factors has to do directly with the foods you eat and the health of your digestive tract. The reason is simple: the gut and the brain have an intimate connection. Michael Gershon, professor of anatomy and cell biology at Columbia University, was the first to claim the existence of what he called the *gut brain* or *second brain*.[6] Properly known as the enteric nervous system (ENS),[7] it resides in the gut, which encompasses all of the organs of digestion, from the esophagus to the anus.

The ENS is one of the main divisions of the autonomic nervous system, and it consists of a system of neurons that governs the function of the gut. In fact, it contains approximately 500 million neurons—as many neurons as the spinal cord—and four times as many glia. As food is digested, the ENS monitors its contents.[8] A thin semipermeable epithelial barrier, which is continuously regenerated by gastrointestinal stem cells,[9] facilitates absorption but also prevents the leakage of essential molecules out of the gut and into the body.[10] All of the functions of digestion, as well as maintaining the integrity of this barrier, are orchestrated by the ENS, including bowel motility, response to sensory stimuli, regulation of blood flow, support of epithelial function, and modulation of immunity. To perform all of these roles, there are at least 14 enteric neuron subtypes that express every neurotransmitter in the CNS.

Virtually every class of neurotransmitter found in the CNS is detectable in the ENS. Yet while the ENS can function without input from the CNS, it does not normally do so. In fact, the brain is more of a receiver than a transmitter with respect to brain–gut communication.[11] Gut-to-brain signaling transmits sensations of nausea, bloating, or satiety, whereas the information sent from the bowel to the CNS could be a determinant of mood. In fact, the vagus nerve, found in the digestive tract, can be stimulated successfully to treat depression and has been demonstrated to improve learning and memory.[12]

Today, we believe that some CNS disorders might relate to the ENS, as dysfunctional gastrointestinal manifestations appear to precede CNS symptoms.[13] Several such disorders with CNS and gastrointestinal manifestations include autism spectrum disorder, Parkinson's disease (PD), and Alzheimer's disease (AD). What's more, studies of autism and neuro-degenerative disorders have shown that the ENS can be both an innocent bystander as well as an active player in CNS disease.

The emergence of well-known neurological viral and bacterial infections as causes of potentially serious gastrointestinal disturbance highlights the importance of the ENS and its connections to the rest of the nervous system.

We also know that early experiments[14] have provided the link between the gut and neuropsychiatric illness. When searching for the greatest source of serotonin in the body, Gershon found that its production was localized to the enteric nervous system. Conventional serotonin-enhancing antidepressants, notably selective serotonin reuptake inhibitors and serotonin–norepinephrine reuptake inhibitors, which have been shown to be effective in the treatment of depression through the stimulation and blockade of various subtypes of 5-hydroxytryptophan (5-HT) receptors, appear to shape the developing brain in even more surprising ways. It is believed that neurodevelopment passes through sensitive periods, during which plasticity allows for genetic and environmental factors to exert indelible influence on the maturation of the organism. In the context of CNS development, such sensitive periods shape the formation of neuro-circuits that mediate, regulate, and control behavior.

YOUR GENETICS AND YOUR MICROBIOMES

The body is colonized by an enormous array of microbes that are collectively called the microbiota or microbiome. Every surface of the body naturally harbors unique microbial communities, called *microbiomes*. These communities of bacteria, viruses, and parasites form as a result of ecological successions where certain microbes adapt to their given niche. Although these microbial communities are relatively resistant to change, factors such as alterations in diet and the administration of antibiotics can result in modifications in microbial community structure.

Science is now coming to understand that we, as human beings, can be thought of as superorganisms that are constantly integrating the identity, function, and immunity of these resident bacteria with our own cells. What's more, our genetics are further influenced by the microbes we are carrying in and on our body and in the human genome. Our innate and adaptive immune systems have developed to deal with these invading organisms. When combined with an underlying genetic vulnerability, and individual differences in exposure timing and host immune responses, it may further explain why some people are more likely to develop medical, neurologic, and neuropsychiatric disorders.

In knowing that the gut is really an immune system for the body, it makes sense that the microbes in your gut and your untreated gastrointestinal problems can influence your genetic predisposition for neurological symptoms. Sampling bacteria and viruses, and registering insults at a very, very early age when they make an impression on your immune system, can contribute to inherent allergies. This is why I-Cubed is increasingly recognized to be caused by the resident microbes that have the capacity to trigger our immune system. The microbiome in the gut has specifically been shown to play an essential role in the establishment of normal immunity, and it is the cause of altered immunity in both the body and the brain. For instance, the axis of communication between the gut and brain, called the mind–gut connection, can be affected by an altered gut microbiome and account for psychiatric symptoms including balance disturbance, headache, neuropsychiatric illness, mood and/ or anxiety disorders, behavioral disorders, attention deficit, intellectual disability, and neuropathy.

Two research studies published simultaneously in the journal *Science*[15] and *Nature*[16] paved the way for two large-scale genomic projects to investigate the human microbiome. Such studies revealed the enormous diversity of microbial flora. There are at least 160 species in the large intestine alone in any given individual. The composition of a person's gastrointestinal flora may not be as unique as a thumbprint, but it is certainly specialized based upon an individual's environmental influences and health status.

THE ROLE OF STRESS ON MICROBIOMES

Physical and psychological stress can disrupt a microbiome's homeostasis and significantly change the community structure, ultimately affecting autoimmunity. Again, this is particularly evident in the gut's microbiome. Such effects are most evident early in life, where both stress and the microbiota are linked to early brain development.[17] We also believe that the origins of adult disease can be traced to the adverse influences early in development, such as poor nutrition, infection, or stress.[18] Neurodevelopment is sensitive to a mother's stresses during pregnancy and is now thought to result in potentially long-lasting behavioral consequences.[19]

The microbiome is an emerging candidate as a potential mediator of stress-induced disease, causing alterations in the HPA axis and subsequent immune function. Any imbalances to an organism homeostasis elicit a complex stress response that involves the coordinated activation of functionally overlapping neuroendocrine and autonomic systems. These critical systems can be triggered by infectious, immunological, and emotional stresses, which then release the stress hormone cortisol into the bloodstream. The activity of the HPA axis is regulated by multiple afferent sympathetic, parasympathetic, and limbic circuits (e.g., amygdala, hippocampus, and medial prefrontal cortex) innervating either directly or indirectly the hypothalamus.

The hypothalamus integrates converging stimulatory (catecholaminergic, glutamatergic, and serotonergic) or inhibitory (GABA-ergic) inputs, and thus exerts control over the HPA axis.[20] Corticotropin-releasing hormone (CRH) and arginine vasopressin released in the portal circulation of the anterior pituitary gland triggers the secretion of the adrenocorticotrophic hormone into the bloodstream by the pituitary gland and induces the production and systemic release of cortisol by the adrenal gland cells.[21] It is believed that brain plasticity and normal brain function during periods of stress depend upon an adequate level of cortisol and other brain hormones.

While activation of the HPA axis is essential for survival during stress, chronic exposure to stress hormones predisposes the individual to psychological, metabolic, and immune alterations. Thus prompt termination of the stress response is essential to prevent negative effects of inappropriate levels of circulating CRH and corticosteroids. The termination of CRH transcription, which is a critical step in this process, is important in healthy neurodevelopment throughout the lifespan.

There is clear evidence that increases in corticosteroids and central levels of CRH can have damaging effects and contribute to depression, anxiety, neurodegeneration, and immune and metabolic disorders.

Altered sympathetic adrenal activity has a major role in the pathophysiology underlying common human diseases. The autonomic disorder orthostatic hypotension leads to an abrupt fall in systolic blood pressure upon standing or tilting. This is due to disturbed sympathetic neural reflexes initiated by baroreceptors that fail to increase peripheral vascular resistance. It is the failure to release the approximately two-fold needed increase in plasma norepinephrine from sympathetic postganglionic neurons that underlies this disturbed reflex.

If you are an individual instead with POTS, you may have an unknown source of anxiety and stress that is resulting from an altered autonomic function. In a sense, you are hardwired to have an accelerated heart rate, even when stress is not a factor. It may occur when you are simply standing up in front of a crowd and a vicious cycle ensues with the feeling that your heart is pounding in your throat rendering you speechless. So while you might have thought your feelings of dizziness were caused by the anxiety of having to speak in front of a crowd, it may simply be your neurobiology. This is also why other people in your family may also experience unrelenting episodes of tachycardia or labile blood pressure or often feel exhausted.

A NEW GENETIC RELATIONSHIP: THE RCCX THEORY

Your precise genetic makeup, and the way the immune system reacts, may be causing a complex of symptoms that we're just beginning to recognize as a syndrome or disease. For instance, there has been recent interest in the genetic entity termed RCCX that expresses four linked HLA genes. It is related to a condition known as congenital adrenal hyperplasia (CAH), which is a disturbance in women who develop hirsutism and bone problems. The R stands for one obsolete gene. The first C stands for the CYP21A2 gene that encodes 21-hydroxylase, which is mutated in CAH. The next C stands for C4, a complement protein that deals with infections; a deficiency due to genetic disturbance of C4 would make someone less able to deal with infectious exposures. Finally, the X stands for a type of benign joint hypermobility syndrome encoded by the tenascin X (TNXB) gene that provides instructions for making a protein called tenascin-XB. This gene and the protein it encodes plays an important role in organizing and maintaining the structure of connective tissues that supports the body's muscles, joints, organs, and skin. When mutated or deficient, it leads to the syndrome of benign joint hypermobility. Interestingly, women with RCCX are often the ones that become dancers, ballerinas, or cheerleaders because they have such hypermobile joints. Yet as they get older, they get stiffer, or they have joint problems. And many such patients present with later POTS. Others have joint hypermobility that leads to shoulder and hip dislocations. Still others develop joint pain and burning sensations that we refer to as painful small fiber neuropathy, which is related to peripheral nerve dysfunction.

This theory was first identified by Dr. Sharon Meglathery, a board-certified internist and psychiatrist. Meglathery developed Ehlers-Danlos syndrome (EDS), which according to the Mayo Clinic is a group of inherited disorders that affect connective tissues, including the skin, joints, and blood vessel walls. People who have EDS usually have overly flexible joints and stretchy, fragile skin.

In the context of this diagnosis, Meglathery also developed mast cell activation, POTS, raised intracranial pressure, chronic fatigue syndrome, and a host of other disabling syndromes in 2009.[22] Her quest to uncover the cause of her own health crisis led her to discover the link between these overlapping syndromes: a genetic neuropsychiatric marker, which she dubbed CAPS, which also predicts a higher risk of chronic illness. Her RCCX theory explains the co-inheritance of a wide range of overlapping chronic medical conditions in individuals and families, ranging from EDS/benign joint hypermobility, autoimmune diseases, chronic fatigue syndrome (CFS), psychiatric conditions, autism, as well as a sensitivity to Lyme disease, fibromyalgia, toxic mold, Epstein-Barr virus (EBV) infection, mast cell activation syndrome (MCAS), POTS, and others. She also believes that this gene is related to a predisposition toward brilliance, gender fluidity, autistic features, and stress vulnerability, as well as the entire spectrum of psychiatric conditions (other than schizophrenia which can be co-inherited).

With its high number of immune system genes that allow for enhanced coordination of expression, RCCX has rapidly diversified by recombination and sequence exchanges rendering it a highly evolutionarily adaptable, and therefore highly conserved, genetic locus. Epigenetic changes have likely been important in the RCCX module and in conferring highly divergent haplotypes, polymorphisms, and phenotypes across human populations.

The *C4*, *CYP21A2*, and *TNXB* genes of the RCCX module have been extensively studied in autoimmune disease and connective tissue disorders. Extending genetic analysis from a causative single gene perspective to the whole RCCX module in relation to phenotype is of great importance. For example, investigators find that patients with congenital adrenal hyperplasia have greater C4 gene copy number variation, which plays an important role in generating necessary variation in the population, and mutation-specific associations that may be protective for autoimmune disease.[23]

Practically speaking, however, recognizing one disorder in the RCCX module in a given individual enables the clinician to postulate the existence or propensity for one of the other genetically encoded or highly associated disorders such as POTS, MCAS, CFS, and neuropsychiatric illness, often in association with EDS/benign joint hypermobility. In addition, as many of the associated illness are chronic in nature, RCCX has become synonymous with the propensity for chronic disease.

Meet Stella

Stella was a 38-year-old writer with joint hypermobility since age 8. She had recurrent childhood strep infections and gastrointestinal complaints, and developed symptoms of depression in her teens. She had two episodes of major depressive disorder, both with suicidal ideation at age 18 and 24 years. Both Stella and her mother are carriers of the *BRCA2* gene for breast cancer, yet neither has developed it. However, Stella developed hypothyroidism and gained 40 pounds. She has had orthostatic dizziness, burning, numbness, tingling, cognitive and mood disturbances, and daily chronic headache since 2015.

By the time she came to see me, Stella's psychiatrist attributed her mood disturbance to depression and anxiety. My examination showed distal sensory loss, weakness, imbalance, and incoordination. There was mild cervical paraspinal tenderness. Electromyography and nerve conduction studies showed a peripheral neuropathy. My autonomic studies showed low blood pressure to account for dizziness, headache, lightheadedness, and heaviness of the arms. Left calf and thigh epidermal nerve fiber studies showed significantly low density in the calf with normal thigh density. Although she was recently treated for tick-borne disease, Lyme serology was non-reactive and there were no circulating autoantibodies apart from anti-thyroidal antibody. Fluorodeoxyglucose positron emission tomography of the brain fused with magnetic resonance imaging and volumetric analysis, also called Neuro-Quant, showed hypometabolism of the brain in discrete areas.

These findings were consistent with distal acquired demyelinating neuropathy, painful small fiber neuropathy, and orthostatic hypotension, cognitive and early onset neuropsychiatric disturbances combined with posterior cerebral hypometabolism. This was all in the setting of long-standing gastrointestinal complaints, benign joint hypermobility, major depressive disorder (MDD), benign breast cancer 2 (*BRCA2*) genetics, food sensitivity and allergies, and treated tick-borne disease exposure. To that was added endocrinopathy manifested by early ovarian failure, acquired hypothyroidism, and reduced serum complement. One might say that this is an extraordinary number of coincidences, but I would venture to say that each one contributed to her neurological illness, and failure to address even the most minute or seemingly irrelevant aspect might have led to an incomplete recovery. Thus our treatment strategy was to address each problem individually with the knowledge and confidence that there is a supreme unifying aspect of genetics, post-infectious autoimmunity, and other allergic triggers.

II

TAPES: A 5-STEP ACTION PLAN

5

Test for an Autoimmune Disturbance

You now have a firm understanding of the underlying causes for your illness. This includes the way both the brain and the immune system works, and how one affects the other. You can also see how I-Cubed, your genetics, and a combination of the two may be the culprit. This background information is necessary, but the goal of this book is to help you feel better.

There are a number of steps that can be taken from the moment of suspicion of the diagnosis of an autoimmune disorder involving the nervous system. Preempting this process would have been unthinkable a decade ago, but medical science has paved the way for holistic anti-inflammatory brain health programs focusing on optimal brain and body nutrition, integrating exercise, conscious mental health, and effective immune modulation.

The first step is identifying exactly what your symptoms are and then determining if you are suffering from an autoimmune issue that is causing brain health problems. To that end, I have developed an early detection and treatment model that is based on a simple 5-step plan that can help both adults and children reverse their brain health issues as well as their physical health by resetting the immune system. My protocol will give you a new approach toward investigating your problem, point you toward appropriate further testing to confirm your suspicions, and ultimately give you the therapeutic tools to restore health and reverse disease. Some treatment options require medical supervision; others do not.

You can easily remember the protocol by the acronym TAPES:

- *Test* for the most likely autoimmune disturbance, and discover how a specific autoimmune response may be affecting brain health.
- *Apply* immune-modulating therapies (under a doctor's care) that will address both the immune response and changes to brain health.
- *Participate* in the most effective behavioral/therapeutic options to reduce stress and reverse fatigue, anxiety, depression, and memory loss.
- *Eat and exercise* to restore brain health, alleviate pain, and enhance the immune system.
- *Survey* your home for chemical exposures, and remove mold and heavy metals that can stand in the way of a full recovery.

This chapter is the first step in my action plan: the art of medical diagnosis. It features an easy-to-follow self-assessment that you can use right at home to help you determine what is causing your (or a loved one's) brain health symptoms.

The purpose of this assessment is twofold. Beyond the obvious benefit of determining your symptoms, it also provides a place for you to record them before you see a doctor. Your doctor can be a full partner in getting you back to health, yet the hard work of arriving at a correct diagnosis starts with your own investigative skills.

THE PAINFUL DRAMA OF MISDIAGNOSIS

I once had a patient, Jessie, who came to see me in her senior year of high school. By that time, she had been cutting herself for two years and had gone through every type of therapy. Her parents were completely perplexed: her mother told me that Jessie's behavioral change from an optimistic, hardworking student who was destined for the Ivies turned sullen with the flick of a switch. None of the doctors or therapists she had seen had suggested medical testing, even though she didn't respond at all to classic depression medication.

My job was to figure out what Jessie's problems were and where they came from. Then, I could give her the right tools that would help her get back to a more normal state. When she came to see me, we immediately ordered brain imaging and found that her results were not only highly abnormal, but the likely cause of her depression. No amount of talk or behavioral therapy was going to resolve Jessie's brain illness.

I cannot say strongly enough how critical proper testing is to finding the right diagnosis. Any patient could present like Jessie, as chronically depressed, but unless you know why the depression isn't lifting, you can't understand where it is coming from. So many people have been seeing a therapist for 10 years and not getting better. Or maybe they've been on antidepressants for 5 years and not getting better. These so-called hopeless cases may turn out to be something entirely different once you correctly examine the brain and body.

Here's a list of classic brain health symptoms that are very often misdiagnosed, and may be related to I-Cubed:

- Attention deficit hyperactivity disorder
- Agitation
- Anxiety
- Brain fog
- Depersonalization
- Depression
- Fatigue
- Inability to feel
- Lassitude
- Lethargy
- Loss of interest in life, job, spouse, children, or family
- Obsessions and compulsions
- Paranoia
- Parasitosis
- Promiscuity
- Psychosis
- Post-traumatic stress disorder
- Rage
- Somatization (attributing symptoms falsely to mental illness)
- Malingering
- Tourette's syndrome of tics and OCD

THE I-CUBED BATTERY

The following questionnaires focus on the primary mechanisms of I-Cubed: infections, pain, neuropathies, cancer, incidences of traumatic stress, as well as the early warning signs of many autoimmune diseases. The battery is comprised of three unique tests to help diagnose an autoimmune brain health issue. The first test will clearly show how an underlying illness may cause brain symptoms including fatigue, forgetfulness, anxiety, depression, poor attention, loss of memory, and more. Identifying the autoimmune component is critical for proper diagnosis, because in almost all instances, if there is a diagnosis of an infectious autoimmune process, such as Lyme disease, there may also be co-infections: additional infectious diseases carried by the same tick that are transmitted at the time of the tick bite. Or when a primary allergic and autoimmune disorder such as Celiac disease is associated with another autoimmune process affecting a different part of the body or hormonal system, such as Hashimoto's thyroiditis or diabetes.

The second test will allow you to see if there is a likelihood of an underlying inherited illness, and if there is, to confirm your findings with accurate genetic testing. The third test will help you determine if your minor head injury is unknowingly a concussion, or if you had one, to see if its effects are still active.

These tests are the best and least invasive ways for you to figure out and manage your symptoms: the results will direct you to the appropriate chapters in the book for specific treatments.

You will need a journal or notebook to record your results. Then take this journal and this book to your doctor and share what you've learned.

TEST I: DETERMINE YOUR SYMPTOMS

You are at risk for a nervous system and systemic autoimmune disturbance if you have symptoms including *memory loss, lack of focus, weakness, incoordination, pain, and lightheadedness*. Remember, systemic inflammation accompanies a variety of allergic, autoimmune, infectious, toxic, and metabolic brain processes, traumatic brain injury, and neurological hereditary disorders. Even low-grade inflammation promotes disturbance of the blood–brain barrier (BBB). When this occurs, brain cells secrete inflammatory molecules called cytokines that disturb normal functioning leading to a range of cognitive and neuropsychiatric manifestations. Disruption of the BBB causes entry of plasma components including cytokines, inflammatory cells, and immune T- and B-cells with a memory of the triggering event, as well as any circulating pathogenic antibodies derived from an existing systemic illness. These initiate varying degrees of reversible brain dysfunction. The following test will help you connect the dots from your symptoms to possible causes.

Step One: Identify Your Symptoms

Directions:

In your journal, write down each item that describes you, your habits, and how you feel. Each answer is worth one point. Add up the points in each category and write the subtotal in your journal.

Infection:

1. I take antibiotics almost every month for either strep throat or ear infections.
2. I know I have an infectious illness like strep throat, Lyme disease, or one of its co-infections because my thinking becomes foggy or people tell me I'm behaving strangely.
3. I have sinus headaches that don't respond to over-the-counter medications.
4. I'm an outdoors person; my property and home is in or near the woods.
5. Certain medications make me feel forgetful, irritable, or depressed, and give me stomach pains and/or bladder issues.
6. I have, or have had, a mold issue in my home.
7. I have had déjà vu episodes or other attacks I thought might be seizures.
8. I suffer with fever, chills, fatigue, low appetite, and muscle aches.
9. I have non-healing sores and recurrent rashes.
10. It takes a long time for me to fight off an infection, heal a wound, or get over a cold.

Subtotal:

Neuropathic Pain:

1. I experience burning skin sensations.
2. I do not like the feeling of my clothes on my skin and am sensitive to touch.
3. My legs are restless at night in bed.
4. I have lightheadedness when I stand up quickly.
5. I have chronically low blood pressure readings.
6. I have frequent heart palpitations.
7. My hands or feet are uncomfortable in the cold.
8. I have numbness or tingling in my hands and feet.
9. Weak muscles prevent me from exercising and even going to work.
10. I have frequent night sweats.

Subtotal:

Autoimmunity:

1. I was chronically ill in infancy or childhood.
2. I have stomach rumbling and frequent flatulence.
3. I have been taking oral or intravenous antibiotics for longer than a year.
4. I have digestive problems when I eat milk and wheat products.
5. I am a highly allergic person and carry an EpiPen in case of anaphylaxis.
6. I had asthma as a child and even now sometimes wheeze.
7. I once had butterfly rash on my face or a bullseye rash on my body.
8. I bruise easily and have a mottled appearance of the skin.
9. I have noted stiff arthritic-like pains, swelling, or joint deformities.
10. One or more relatives suffer from an autoimmune disease.

Subtotal:

Neurocognitive:

1. I have a sudden loss of memory.
2. I cannot multitask anymore.
3. I have to make lists, or I will forget or confuse appointments.
4. I have difficulty with complex tasks like driving.
5. I have been unfocused at work or school.
6. I have been told that I'm not as sharp as I used to be.
7. I have made frequent mistakes at work or in school.
8. I find it hard to finish a task.
9. I need to take frequent naps or take breaks during the day.
10. I'm drinking more coffee and eating more than I used to help me with energy and focus.

Subtotal:

Neurobehavioral:

1. I feel unmotivated.
2. I obsess over minor details.
3. I have ritualistic behaviors.
4. I spend a lot of time in my bedroom or at home.
5. I have been crying and getting upset at people more than usual.

6. I drink to calm myself down; I use street drugs or medications to stabilize my mood.
7. I have uncontrollable movements in my hands or feet.
8. I make weird noises.
9. I am sensitive to noise or light.
10. I have been told that I don't communicate well with others.

Subtotal:

General Health:

1. I have noticed more frequent urination.
2. I have diarrhea and constipation.
3. I cannot exercise like I used to.
4. I have brain fog.
5. I am overly sensitive to the temperature around me.
6. I have had a change in libido or sexual performance.
7. My hair, nails, or skin have changed.
8. I have recently lost or gained weight without trying.
9. I have unrefreshing sleep.
10. I have chronic fatigue.

Subtotal:

Interpretation:

1. If you have five or more symptoms from the categories of *autoimmunity, neurocognitive,* or *neurobehavioral,* OR a total score of 15 or more from those categories, then your brain health changes may be linked to an autoimmune brain disorder. If you have five or more symptoms from the categories of *infection* or *general health,* OR a total score of 10 or more from those categories, then you likely have a chronic infectious disorder and post-infectious autoimmunity that is affecting your thinking and behavior.
2. If you have five or more symptoms from the category of *neuropathic pain,* then you likely have painful small fiber neuropathy which, like brain auto-immunity, is another source of nervous system damage.
3. If you have five or more symptoms from only the *neurobehavioral* or *neurocognitive* categories than you have a neuropsychological issue and should

be under the care of a neurologist and a licensed psychiatrist or therapist. The rest of the chapters in part II should be particularly helpful, and a great place to start reversing your symptoms. Chapter 7 will be invaluable in helping you decide which types of mental health therapies are best for you.

Step Two: Categorize Your Symptoms

As you've learned, neurological disorders can be conveniently divided into those that lead to brain and spinal cord, or central nervous system (CNS) dysfunction; those that affect the large and small peripheral nerves, and lead to peripheral nervous system (PNS) or neuropathic disturbances; and others that affect autonomic nervous system (ANS) pathways that modulate vital signs and involuntary organ function. Some symptoms will fall neatly into one of these categories and be unmistakable for a given disorder, and therefore yield the answer in short order, while others may be vague enough that they straddle several categories at once.

These three systems, CNS, PNS and ANS, are schematically shown as a Venn diagram, with separate yet overlapping circles. In Figure 5.1, the upper left hand corner represents the CNS, consisting of the brain and spinal cord. Motor neurons of the brain send their axons into the spinal cord to innervate the arms and legs thereby allowing you to perform coordinated movements. Other neurons in brain's temporal (limbic) lobe control your emotions, while frontal areas oversee executive functioning and planning. Thus, typical symptoms of CNS disorders include neurocognitive issues of fatigue, headaches, brain fog, memory loss, mood and psychiatric symptoms, as well as, incoordination and gait difficulty.

The PNS depicted in the right hand corner contains large nerve fibers insulated with a myelin sheath, and small unmyelinated nerve fibers. The large nerve fibers are the width of a linguini strand. The small nerve fibers, typically found in the skin, are microscopic. Typical symptoms of PNS disorders include pain, sensory loss, numbness, tingling, weakness and muscle wasting.

The ANS situated in the bottom circle regulates bodily functions, from the secretion of glands to the concerted regulation of multiple organ functions body wide. Vascular channels and nerve fibers connect the brain's hypothalamus to the pituitary gland and the latter, directly to the our major organs, through an intricate network of autonomic nerve fibers and ganglia that regulate vital signs, postural reflexes, secretory glandular function, and overall body homeostasis. Typical symptoms of ANS disorders include hypotension, palpitations, sweating, loss of hair, and redness or paleness of the skin.

You can use this diagram to start to categorize your symptoms. As you enter your symptoms, see if you can rank them in the order they appeared. You may be surprised to see for yourself how your symptoms can be filed into each circle. What's more, you may see that the progression begins in the most vulnerable aspects of the nervous system. Many patients tell me that their earliest symptoms are due to concomitant involvement of small nerve fibers in the skin whose terminal branches have both sensory and autonomic functions. Their involvement causes numbness or burning sensations, and lightheadedness and palpitations and sometimes symptoms of panic. This is often followed by weakness due to larger nerve fibers of the PNS, and eventually, CNS issues like brain fog and mood disturbances. I believe that symptoms progress in this fashion with the last one in the CNS because it takes time for antibodies and the inflammatory response to disrupt the BBB. What's more, when symptoms are left untreated, they become more severe over time.

Draw the following image in your journal, and fill in your symptoms. Give the results of this test and your Venn diagram to your doctor. From here, they will be able to order the appropriate testing to confirm your findings.

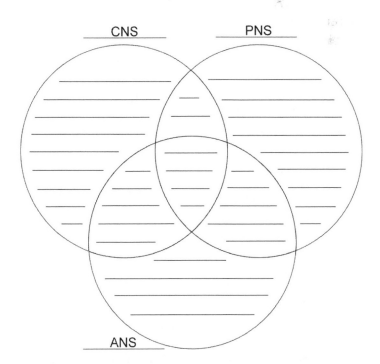

TEST II: YOUR GENETIC PROFILE

The following symptoms are commonly associated with specific neurological genetic disorders.

Review these symptoms and write the ones you are experiencing in your journal, and then show the results and this list to your doctor:

- Joint hypermobility (Ehlers-Danlos syndrome): hyperextensible joints
- Gluten (wheat) sensitivity (Celiac disease): bloating after eating food with wheat
- Hammer toes (Charcot-Marie Tooth neuropathology): deformed toes
- Postural dizziness and orthostatic hypotension with tachycardia (inherited dysautonomia): lightheadedness upon standing
- Staring spells, convulsions, and automatisms (genetic forms of epilepsy): spells of altered consciousness with or without muscle shaking
- Stiff neck/torticollis (genetic dystonia): fixed postures of the hands or feet
- Vocal and motor tics, obsessive compulsive disorders (Tourette syndrome): uncontrolled vocal utterances and motor movements accompanied by obsessive rituals like hand washing.
- Muscle weakness (genetic myopathy or muscular dystrophy): arm or leg weakness
- Rigidity and stiffness (Parkinson's disease): shuffling gait and hand tremor
- Memory loss and dementia (Alzheimer's disease): forgetfulness and mood change
- Proptosis and hyperactive (Grave's disease and Hashimoto's thyroiditis): bulging of eyes and prominent stare
- Frequent infections and sore throats (common variable immune deficiency)

TEST III: TESTING FOR CONCUSSION

A concussion, or mild traumatic brain injury, results from a blow to the head and disrupts normal brain functioning immediately; symptoms can last for a period of up to months or even a year. The motor, cognitive, emotional, and psychosocial consequences of concussion can be devastating, whether short or long term, with rapid deterioration of a domain of normal mental abilities and independent function. The associated symptoms and neurobehavioral changes can mimic the psychiatric manifestation of a psychiatric disorder with prominent mood changes, difficulty adjusting to daily routine, confusion, depression, and even psychotic symptoms such as a fear of walking through a doorway or being injured.

A concussive head injury can cause localized and immediate damage both at the area of impact as well as in much broader areas of cerebral functions, because the injury itself can damage the BBB. As you've learned in the previous chapters, the BBB is the protective cellular lining that covers the brain, and when it is intact it prevents infections and inflammation from entering. However, when the barrier is compromised, the autoimmune response can affect brain health secondary to the concussion. In this way, a concussion can create an autoimmune response leading to symptoms. You will learn more about this in chapter 13[1] but for now, you can see how the two types of brain insults, one traumatic and the other post-concussive and potentially inflammatory, are related.

This last quiz[2] will help you recognize if you or a loved one has suffered a concussive head injury. Review these symptoms and write the ones you are experiencing in your journal, and then show the results and this list to your doctor:

- Any period of loss of consciousness, including difficulty awakening, or unresponsiveness to arousal
- Vacant stare: a befuddled facial expression
- Delayed verbal and motor responses: slow to answer questions or follow instructions
- Confusion and inability to focus attention: easily distracted and unable to follow through with normal activities of daily living such as plans to meet friends or tune into a favorite television show or radio broadcast
- Disorientation: walking in the wrong direction, unaware of time, date, and place
- Slurred or incoherent speech, or making disjointed or incomprehensible statements
- Observable incoordination, including stumbling, inability to walk in a straight line
- Emotions out of proportion to circumstances: distraught, crying for no apparent reason
- Low-grade persistent headache
- Dizziness or vertigo
- Lack of awareness of surroundings

- Nausea or vomiting
- Light-headedness
- Inattention and impaired concentration
- Memory disturbance
- Easy fatigability
- Irritability and low frustration tolerance
- Intolerance of bright lights
- Difficulty focusing vision
- Intolerance of loud noises and/or tinnitus
- Anxiety and depressed mood
- Sleep disturbance
- Memory deficits exhibited by repeatedly asking the same question that has already been answered, or inability to memorize and recall 3/3 words or 3/3 objects in 5 minutes

If you have had a head injury with or without loss of consciousness and checked off five or more symptoms, read chapter 13 to see more detailed information on concussions.

BEST PRACTICES FOR PREPARING FOR YOUR DOCTOR

The next step is choosing the right physician who can corroborate your findings. I am a strong advocate for starting with your internist or general practitioner, as they know your health history best. However, if your brain health is not improving quickly, you will eventually need to see a neurologist.

You are fully within your rights as a patient to share in the investigative experience of your illness as a medical detective. As a doctor, I fully appreciate it when a patient comes in prepared for our initial consultation. Yet more often than not my patients, or their parents, may be so stressed, overwhelmed, or just feeling so poorly that they cannot adequately organize and present their thoughts or their own findings. I can't tell you how many times a patient walks into my office with an overflowing folder or a six-inch pile of paper and states, *"I know I have the answer here somewhere, but I can't find it."* This often results from their illness and the way it disturbs their thinking processes.

Here's a secret: the most organized patients really do get the most optimal care, so do your best to stay focused. I also see plenty of people who take the time to organize their materials, research, and reports. In fact, dumping unorganized notes onto a doctor's lap makes all of your hard work virtually useless. Unless your doctor can do something with it, that is to say they can go through the records carefully and translate it into useful information, it becomes even more challenging to come up with a diagnosis compared to when a patient does not do any personal investigation. That's why I've created this assessment. It can provide you with the beginning framework for your detective work.

Bring this assessment to your next doctor's visit, even if you are seeing the same doctor you have always been using. Your results will highlight the most likely metabolic, inflammatory autoimmune, genetic, degenerative, or infectious causes, alone or in combination, and yield compelling insights for your doctor as to the location within the nervous system where your problem resides.

It's also absolutely worth the time to write out a narrative of your medical history in your own words, including how you feel right now. This narrative should include the progression of your symptoms, complete with dates and any recollections you may have of when certain symptoms emerged, and how they have progressed over time. Lastly, organize any additional research you've done, as well as any testing results or medical paperwork you may already have.

A savvy physician will be intrigued and not necessarily put off by your efforts. The history provides a window to the type of ailment you may be experiencing and will help the doctor determine whether it falls into the category of a metabolic, inflammatory autoimmune, genetic, degenerative, or infectious illness. From there, the doctor can do a more thorough examination and order subsequent testing to confirm the problem.

I like to tell prospective patients or their parents to put their information onto a single electronic medical record resource that can easily be shared with me. The best options are forwarding electronic files before our office visit or handing me a thumb drive or USB that I can easily plug into my computer so that I can download their records.

Having electronic medical records underscores the importance of staying with a team of doctors who are all associated with a single institution or hospital. This makes the transfer of information from one doctor to another relatively easy. What's more, all your doctors will be able to see all the data that's available, and then provide the best care.

MEETING WITH YOUR DOCTOR

1. Confirm the date and time of your appointment with the office secretary and ask for his or her name to establish a friendly rapport. These people are the "gatekeepers" to a well-run office, and your quality of care can easily be influenced by your relationships with them.

2. Invite a trusted friend or close relative to come with you to the visit to boost your confidence, take notes, and remind you of questions to ask your doctor.

3. Bring extra copies of records and any previous scans that you can leave with the doctor's office.

4. Provide your doctor with your previous health history and any additional information if you have allergies or are currently taking medications. Typically, the doctor's office will provide you with a checklist for this, but if not, be prepared to create one.

5. Dress casually with loose fitting clothes that can easily be removed if necessary for your examination. A doctor's visit is not a fashion contest, and a humble presentation makes a better impression than an ostentatious one.

6. Bring along a body spray in case you arrive sweating, and gym shorts if you are typically uncomfortable in either a paper or tight-fitting medical gown.

7. Ask the doctor for visual images of the diagnosis if you don't understand their explanations.

8. Make sure that your doctor reviews each of the five pillars of a comprehensive diagnosis (known as a *differential diagnosis*): are there *metabolic, autoimmune, genetic*, and *drug-induced* causes of illness, *alone or in combination*.

THE IMPORTANCE OF MEDICAL TESTING

A doctor can confirm your findings and evaluate the presence of an autoimmune disorder and its effect on the nervous system through a wide variety of tests.

The screening tests that point to problems in the CNS look for abnormalities in brain structure, perfusion or metabolism. This can be assessed by magnetic resonance imaging (MRI) of the brain and the total (cervical, thoracic, and lumbosacral) spine. If you are claustrophobic, ask if you can do the imaging in an open unit, but keep in mind that those machines are less sensitive than closed machines. An MRI will show the brain's structure, including demyelinating white matter changes typical of demyelinating diseases, migraines, and Lyme disease. It will also show atrophy or a shrinking of the cortical gray matter structure more typical of autoimmune encephalitis and Alzheimer's.

CNS abnormalities can also be found using one of two types of computed tomographic radiotracer scans. The first is known as SPECT, which stands for single photon emission computerized tomography. A SPECT scan is considered a nuclear imaging test, which means it uses a radioactive substance and a special camera to create three-dimensional pictures. When looking at the brain, it measures areas that are more active or less active, and can detect abnormal cerebral blood flow and the integrity of the BBB.

A third scan, and second computed tomographic option, for CNS abnormalities is a metabolic scan, which can determine how the brain is functioning from a metabolic tissue standpoint. This is typically done using a PET scan, which stands for positron emission tomography. PET imaging uses small amounts of a tagged radioactive tracer that is chemically incorporated into the metabolism of the organs it is studying, such as the brain. The most common approach for studying brain metabolism is to employ radioactive [18]fluorodeoxyglucose or FDG. The tracer then emits radiation as glucose is metabolized, and the intensity of metabolism is recorded as a signal by the scanner using digital pictures Areas that are low in metabolism (hypometabolic) due to injury can be separated from areas of high metabolism (hypermetabolic) characteristic of a seizure focus. This technology readily separates dementia due to depression (pseudodepression) from Alzheimer's. PET combined with body CT can also be used to screen for an early underlying cancer as the latter will light up as a hypermetabolic area in the organ where it is found.

The combination of brain SPECT and PET fused with MRI (PET/MRI) provides useful complimentary measures of blood flow to areas of the brain compared to its metabolic demand for glucose and other nutrients. Together, these tests constitute the sum of the equation of "supply and demand" aspects of the brain at a single point in time in your illness, which is a very useful concept. PET/MRI has become even more useful as a test of hippocampal integrity within the temporal lobe, which is an area associated with neuropsychiatric illness and autoimmune encephalitis.

For patients with isolated CNS involvement, a brain biopsy may be indicated. Timely recognition and treatment of CNS inflammation may improve or even reverse clinical symptoms and prevent secondary brain injury such as in patients with epilepsy and autoimmune encephalitis for whom surgery may be required to either remove the epileptic focus or to examine the brain tissue, further guiding therapy.

The screening tests for the PNS include electrodiagnostic studies of the major peripheral nerves and muscles, termed EMG (electromyography) and nerve conduction studies (NCS). Together, these measure the muscle responses to nerve stimulation, by registering the waveforms that are produced by simple shocks along the arms and legs. Such studies are indispensable in diagnosing peripheral neuropathy and in differentiating the two principal types: demyelinating and axonal. I use the analogy of an ordinary electrical copper wire surrounded by insulation to demonstrate the parts of a nerve fiber that can be targeted by a disease process, and measured by electrodiagnostic studies. Neuropathies associated with altered speed of conduction are typically due to an immune attack of the outer rubbery part of the wire or myelin sheath, and called demyelinating. However, neuropathies due to metabolic, degenerative, or vascular hypoxic diseases that disturb blood flow affect the inner copper wire or axon, and are appropriately called axonal. Unfortunately, this testing has been referred to on the internet as a "torture chamber test," yet I can tell you that it doesn't have to be difficult or uncomfortable. In fact, it is actually an easy, quick, and relatively comfortable test, especially when performed in a doctor's office with calming music. For instance, when I perform this test I warm my patients' feet, dim the lights, play comforting music, and speak in a low tone, making it more like a spa day.

Another useful screening test for the PNS and ANS is a skin biopsy that measures the density or number of microscopic nerve fibers in a millimeter of skin. This is done because the skin is comprised of both small sensory and autonomic nerve fibers. Terminal branches of small sensory fibers innervate receptors in the skin that register pain and temperature and travel along afferent or incoming nerve fibers of the PNS to the brain for conscious appreciation of sensation. Specialized autonomic fibers in the skin innervate sweat glands, hair follicles and blood vessels. This test is useful test to repeat after a course of immunotherapy, along with NCS, because the two together will show rapid gains of therapy within 3 months due to regeneration of nerve fibers. Screening tests for the ANS typically include measurements of heart rate (HR) and systolic blood pressure (BP) in response to rapid and deep breathing, and head-up tilt table testing. ANS disorders can lead to deficient vital signs with postural changes and disturb normal bladder, bowel, and sexual function.

To simply understand the three different types of abnormal tilt table results, I use the objective cutoff of less than one hundred millimeters of mercury BP (< 100 mmHg) as a definition of hypotension; and greater than one hundred beats per minute of HR (> 100 bpm) as the definition of tachycardia. Then, the instance when both BP and HR are > 100 mmHg and 100 bpm with tilting for 5 minutes is indicative of postural orthostatic tachycardia syndrome (POTS), which often produces palpitations and a sense of panic. Situations where both BP and HR are < 100 upon titling indicates instead, primary orthostatic hypotension with an insufficient reflex compensatory HR response. Such patients will often be found to have an underlying autonomic neuropathy and complain of dizziness with abrupt or prolonged standing. However, when the BP is < 100 mmHg and the HR > 100 bpm, this is the likely primary orthostatic hypotension with an adequate reflex compensatory HR response, that may save you from fainting, but produces the uncomfortable sense of palpitations and panic. Each of these disorders is treated differently, and the diagnosis is aided by complementary findings on EMG and NCS and skin biopsy.

Bloodwork panels can screen for infections, metabolic disorders, toxic exposures, vitamin deficiencies, genetic causes, and a host of specific autoimmune diseases. Some conditions can alter one or more parts of the nervous system. For instance, the metabolic illness, diabetes predictably leads to neuropathy (PNS), dysautonomia (ANS), and strokes (CNS), affecting all three categories of the nervous system. So too, can the genetic allergic and autoimmune illness, Celiac disease; and the infectious and post-infectious immune aspects of Lyme disease.

Autoimmune diseases can create autoantibodies that lead to disturbances to the brain without other more revealing symptoms that suggest a disease elsewhere. The Mayo Clinic offers an autoimmune encephalitis panel that can be performed in a single tube of blood to test for all of the known antibodies associated with autoimmune encephalitis.

Basic blood tests include inflammatory markers and autoantibodies. There are also commercially available assays that detect elevated levels of ubiquitin C-terminal hydrolase L1, a neuronal marker of brain injury that rises in the blood after a head injury, including a concussion, due to BBB disruption. Environmental toxic screenings, particularly for mold, lead, and mercury, are important.

Cerebrospinal fluid (CSF) obtained by lumbar puncture may be necessary in patients suspected of harboring meningitis, encephalitis, and non-infectious autoimmune inflmmatory disorders. The procedure should ideally be performed in a hospital setting by a neurologist, anesthesiologist, or radiologist prepared to give you the comfort and confidence you deserve, as well as a place to convalesce for up to three hours lying flat. Remember to drink plenty of fluids before the test, because people who undergo it in a dehydrated state will be at risk for developing a headache.

BOX 5.2

DO I NEED A NEUROQUANT?

Patients will come to me demanding, "the NeuroQuant study" because they have read about it or heard about it on an internet forum or Facebook group. I agree that it is useful in many neuropsychiatric, epileptic, neurocognitive, and degenerative disorders because it looks at the volume of certain areas of the brain in relation to the entire cranial volume occupied by the brain. However, we no longer speak of this testing as NeuroQuant, but a brain scan with "volumetrics," as the software is rapidly changing from NeuroQuant to others.

PROPER TESTING SAVED ANN

Proper testing is one of the key factors to reaching the right diagnosis. I once had a patient named Ann who came to see me with joint pain, fatigue, cramping, muscle pain, and cognitive and behavioral changes. She had a significant déjà vu–like seizure disorder: she often believed she was experiencing something that she had already experienced, when in fact she had not. This is not uncommon among those who suffer from temporal lobe seizures. She also had obsessive-compulsive disorder (OCD), heart palpitations, headaches, and a history of Lyme disease. Her mother told me that Ann had previously been a dynamo: in high school she had been an outgoing cheerleader. Yet when she came to my office, she was extremely bashful and sat through the examination with uncontrollable facial tics. She was also exhibiting problems with basic balance, even though she had relatively normal strength reflexes, and her mental status and cranial nerves were all intact.

Ann's many immune insults, such as recurrent rashes and food allergies, were unusual for this particular 21-year-old woman. This led me to believe that her autoimmune symptoms were stemming from more than just Lyme disease. However, it was quite possible that Lyme disease was sufficient to explain her symptoms. I started the analysis by verifying her Lyme exposure through a screening serology that was positive, however a Western blot analysis suggested only prior Lyme exposure but not active infection. I also did an immune baseline panel, which showed that she had elevated C1q binding, which is an antibody of the complement family of proteins that is drawn to sites of immune complex formation, particularly around blood vessels. Much like the old Road Runner cartoons, when the coyote lights an Acme bomb, the C1q binding assay complex can explode, opening up a hole in the endothelial blood vessel wall and predisposing that area to further injury from leakage of blood and further recruitment of immune mediators.

In order to determine the ultimate cause of her symptoms, we also tested the three major brain systems. Electromyography and nerve conduction studies showed she had a demyelinating neuropathy, which is autoimmune in nature. We also did a skin biopsy for epidermal nerve fiber densities, which showed that microscopic nerve fibers in the skin were decreased, indicating a small fiber neuropathy. Her tilt-table test showed a fall in BP to less than 100 mmHg without a compensatory HR response. A Mayo clinic autoimmune encephalopathy (ENS1) panel revealed an elevated glutamic acid decarboxylase

(GAD) 65 antibody level. A brain PET/MRI performed in 2017 was compared to a new study in 2019 that showed progression in hypometabolism of the frontal, parietal and temporal lobes indicating an evolving immune brain disturbance while being treated with intravenous immune globulin (IVIg) therapy. She was actively deteriorating and manifesting worsened mood and memory. It was necessary to decide whether her deteriorating mental status was due to acute infection or a post-infectious Lyme process, versus GAD65 antibody-mediated autoimmunity.

This dilemma was solved with a lumbar puncture that showed inflammation and protein elevation with a reactive Lyme antibody in the CSF but without Western blot reactivity, or elevation in Borrelia-specific antibodies in the CSF compared to the serum (termed a negative Lyme index) indicating likely inactive infection.

Ann is slowly improving and hopes to return to college. Symptoms and signs of Lyme disease, including suggestive serology and abnormal brain PET/MRI as in Ann's case, have been designated post-treatment Lyme disease syndrome (PTLDS). This appears to be related to non-viable spirochetes or their remnants that persist in the body and fuel a systemic and nervous system immune response long after standard of care treatment.[3] All treating physicians faced with similar patients must decide the appropriate use of antibiotics, IVIg and even biological therapies such as rituximab in this situation. Immune therapy specifically, has the potential to treat both post-infectious and GAD65 antibody-associated immune mechanisms that can improve cognitive and neuropsychiatric symptoms, and brain hypometabolism on PET/MRI.[4]

DON'T WAIT TO SEE YOUR DOCTOR: EARLY DETECTION IS KEY
One of the most important ways we can take better care of ourselves is by proactively attending to our daily health. The truth is that anything that falls short of feeling normal and vibrant means that there may be a short circuit in the nervous system that can be addressed, and hopefully reversed.

For instance, my friend Patricia thought she had a sinus infection. In fact, she gets them all the time, and thought she could address her symptoms the way she always did, with over-the-counter medications. A few days of Sudafed and antihistamines helped clear up her nose, but she was still very tired. It took her a whole week to realize that her constant fatigue was interfering with her work.

Patricia finally went to the doctor, and in the examination room, the nurse asked her how much she weighed, and she laughed when she told me this story. "I told the nurse I weighed 95 pounds, and she looked at me like I was out of my mind. For the life of me, I didn't understand what was happening. Finally, I realized that my brain was not functioning well. I haven't weighed 95 pounds since I was in middle school."

Patricia's story is a classic example of how an infection can impact brain health. Her fatigue and brain fog may be minor symptoms, but they can be easily addressed. The doctor confirmed her suspicions that she did indeed have a sinus infection, and once she started taking her antibiotics, she told me that her brain health symptoms vanished. Had she not gone to the doctor, her sinus infection could have snowballed into more symptoms, including poor attention or poor coordination, which might have led to a much worse outcome.

THE NEXT STEP
Much like high BP, obesity, and other persistent illnesses, autoimmunity needs to be managed daily with an individualized program that works. In the next chapter, you'll learn about the second step of my protocol: applying immune-modulating therapies. This breakthrough treatment is often the difference between living with symptoms and gaining a full recovery.

6

Apply Immune-Modulatory and Pain Therapy

Once you've made a diagnosis of a likely autoimmune disorder, your treatment plan should address both the autoimmune issue and your neurological complaints. The next step is to develop a strategy to address the likeliest mechanisms and the best mode of therapy, using an evidence-based approach.

When we get to this point, my patients often ask me, "Is this therapy going to be a lifetime commitment?" The truth is, any decline in brain health has evolved over a long period of time, and treatment typically takes just as long to resolve these issues. If you can look back and see that your symptoms are relatively recent, you have the best hope for a fast recovery. I've seen people make startling recoveries in six months, and for others, it can take much longer.

Remember, according to the Cleveland Clinic, autoimmune disorders may be viewed as "autoimmune errors" committed by your immune system. Recovery from autoimmune disorders depends on your immune system's ability to correct its own error. In some autoimmune disorders, this occurs in as little as a few weeks, while others take longer. Immune therapy reduces ongoing injury when the organs self-correct the autoimmune error.[1]

As a general rule, in most autoimmune disorders, immunosuppression reduces inflammation and the injury that can occur from inflammation, but it has a minor role in reversing the primary disease process itself. The goal of immune-modulatory therapy is to change the status of the immune system from attack mode to surveillance. The rationale doctors use for choosing a specific treatment depends on many factors, including the severity of the attack, how long it has persisted, and which components of the immune system are involved.

I have focused my career on neuroimmunology—the intersection of neurology and how the immune system affects the nervous system. Through this work, I have developed cutting-edge treatment protocols centered on immune-modulatory therapy (known as intravenous immunoglobulin [IVIg]) that have been adopted by doctors across the country. It has become the most widely employed immune-modulating agent for autoimmune neurological disorders.

Yet IVIg is only one of a host of therapies you can discuss with your doctor, depending on your diagnosis. This chapter explores all of them, so that you can make a good decision, with the help of your doctor, on which treatments will be the most effective. The order of the therapies is listed from least invasive/easiest to acquire (over-the-counter medications) to ones that require special approval from insurance companies and constant supervision from a doctor.

OVER-THE-COUNTER REMEDIES

The least invasive immune therapies that lower inflammation include over-the-counter agents. Non-steroidal anti-inflammatory drugs reduce pain, decrease fever, prevent blood clots, and, in higher doses, decrease inflammation. Side effects depend on the specific drug, but largely include an increased risk of gastrointestinal ulcers and bleeds, heart attack, and kidney disease.

PRESCRIPTION IMMUNOTHERAPIES

The majority of prescription immunotherapies target one or more components of the immune response. For instance, corticosteroids are a class of naturally occurring steroid hormones produced in the adrenal cortex. They are involved in a wide range of physiological processes, including stress response, immune response, and the regulation of inflammation. They are also the most commonly prescribed immunosuppressant medication. They can be administered as a pulse injection of methylprednisolone (Solu Medrol) or hydrocortisone (Solu Cortef) for rapid onset, or in pill form as generic prednisone for sustained periods.

The usefulness of corticosteroids in the treatment of autoimmune disease in general has been appreciated for over 50 years. The beneficial effects of corticosteroids are attributed to a multiplicity of effects on the cell and humoral immune system, but mainly the inhibition of activated T- and B-cells, white blood cells, and inflammatory cytokines at the site of inflammation. Patients receiving long-term corticosteroid therapy should be monitored closely for hypertension, fluid retention, glucose intolerance, cataracts, myopathy, avascular necrosis, infection, gastric and duodenal ulcers, and psychosis, and followed empirically for the need of short-acting insulin coverage as needed. Two serious complications of chronic corticosteroid therapy include osteoporosis and bone fracture. The most susceptible patients, categorized as high in risk, should be offered calcium supplements to prevent bone fractures.

Immunoglobulin (Ig) therapy modulates the proliferation of T-cells, B-cells, and complement activation that are potent driving forces in the immune response, making it the most effective immune modulatory agent. Azathioprine (Imuran) and mycophenolate mofetil (CellCept) suppress both T-cells and B-cells.

The group of biological therapy agents or "biologics" are tailored to specifically target an immune or genetic mediator of disease. They include those that target inflammatory cytokines that perpetuate the immune response. They include etanercept (Enbrel), adalimumab (Humira), and infliximab (Remicade), and others that are even more potent, such as rituximab (Rituxan) that directly targets B-cells. For instance, Rituxan is a monoclonal antibody that depletes B-cells from the circulation. It is used to treat B-cell lymphomas, but it is increasingly employed in the treatment of refractory and severe autoimmune diseases of the central nervous system and peripheral nervous system, as well as systemic vasculitis. Enbrel, Remicade, and Humira derive their immunosuppressant activity by binding to TNF-α. Binding to tumor necrosis factor-alpha reduces the inflammatory response. These medications are generally administered by a healthcare provider as a subcutaneous injection.

The oral antimetabolite agent methotrexate inhibits folate metabolism and is used in the treatment of cancer and rheumatoid arthritis, and is equally effective as corticosteroids in treating autoimmune diseases. However strictly defined, it is not part of the biologics.

The immunosuppressant mycophenolate mofetil or CellCept was originally used to prevent rejection of transplanted organs; however, it is being used increasingly as a corticosteroid-sparing agent in a wide range of systemic and neurological autoimmune diseases. Its immunosuppressant activity derives from its inhibition of purine synthesis. Most experts agree that patients with systemic autoimmune diseases who are poor candidates for corticosteroids and intolerant of Imuran can be treated effectively and safely with long-term CellCept. The following table shows the available therapies for a list of typical primary and secondary autoimmune nervous system disorders.

Table 6.1. Categorization and Treatment of Autoimmune Diseases

Category	Treatment
Systemic Disorders	
A. Genetically Mediated Single Organ Involvement	
1. HLAB27-mediated spondyloarthropathy	TNF inhibitors[1]
2. HLA DQ2/DQ8-mediated Celiac disease	Gluten-free diet, Ig[2,3]
a. Porphyria	Avoid P450 triggers, Heme Rx[4,5]
B. Autoantibody Mediated Multiorgan involvement	
3. Rheumatoid arthritis (bone)	TNF/IL inhibitors[6]
4. Lupus erythematosus (connective tissue)	CS, RTX[7]
5. Thyroiditis (thyroid gland)	Levothyroxine, CS[8]
6. Vasculitis (blood vessels)	Ig/RTX
C. Ill-Defined Pathogenesis	
7. Chronic fatigue syndrome	Supportive[9]
8. Irritable bowel syndrome	Supportive[10]
Nervous System Disorders	
D. Infection-mediated autoimmunity (I-Cubed)	
9. Lyme disease (PNS, CNS, ANS)	Antibiotics/Ig[11]
10. PANDAS	
a. Group A beta hemolytic strep infection	Antibiotics/Ig/PE[12]
11. PANS	
b. Bacteria, viruses, parasites	Antibiotics/Ig/PE
E. Toxin-Related Pathogenesis	
a. Mycotoxins	Experimental[13,14]
b. Heavy metals	Chelation[15]
F. Primary Autoimmunity	
12. Autoimmune encephalitis (specific antibodies)	
a. Antibodies against S Ag (NMDA, VGKC)	Ig, PE, RTX[16]
b. Antibodies against I Ag (GAD65)	Ig, PE, RTX[16]
13. Primary CNS vasculitis	Ig, RTX[17,18]

Category	Treatment
G. Non-Specific Autoimmunity Related to BBB Disruption	
a. Concussion	Supportive[19]
b. Hashimoto encephalopathy	CS[20]
H. Degenerative Illness with Autoimmune Modifiers	
c. Alzheimer's disease (brain cortex)	Experimental[21]
d. Parkinson's disease (subcortical gray matter)	Dopamine agonists[22]

Abbreviations: ANS, autonomic nervous system; BBB, blood–brain barrier; CNS, central nervous system; CS, corticosteroids; GAD, glutamic acid decarboxylase; HLA, human leukocyte antigen; I Ag, intracellular antigen; Ig, immunoglobulin; IL, interleukin; NMDA, n-methyl D-aspartate antibody; NSAID, non-steroidal anti-inflammatory drug; PE, plasma exchange; PNS, peripheral nervous system; RTX, rituximab; S Ag, surface antigen; TNF, tumor necrosis factor; VGKC, voltage gated potassium channel.

1. Her M, Kavanaugh A. Treatment of spondyloarthropathy: the potential for agents other than TNF inhibitors. Curr Opin Rheumatol 2013;25(4):455–59.
2. Schuppan D, Zimmer K-P. The diagnosis and treatment of Celiac disease. Deutsches Ärzteblatt International 2013;110(49):835–46.
3. Younger DS. The human microbiome and I-Cubed: a modern medical paradigm. World Journal of Neuroscience 2016;6:260–86.
4. Pischik E, Kauppinen R. An update of clinical management of acute intermittent porphyria. The Application of Clinical Genetics 2015;8:201–14.
5. Younger DS, Tanji K. Demyelinating neuropathy in genetically confirmed acute intermittent porphyria. Muscle Nerve 2015;52(5):916–17.
6. Shetty A, Hanson R, Korsten P, et al. Tocilizumab in the treatment of rheumatoid arthritis and beyond. Drug Design, Development and Therapy 2014;8:349–64.
7. Schwartz N, Goilav B, Putterman C. The pathogenesis, diagnosis and treatment of lupus nephritis. Current Opinion in Rheumatology 2014;26(5):502–09.
8. Vaidya B, Harris PE, Barrett P, Kendall-Taylor P. Corticosteroid therapy in Riedel's thyroiditis. Postgraduate Medical Journal 1997;73(866):817–19.
9. Rowe PC, Underhill RA, Friedman KJ, et al. Myalgic encephalomyelitis/chronic fatigue syndrome diagnosis and management in young people: a primer. Frontiers in Pediatrics 2017;5:121.
10. Soares RL. Irritable bowel syndrome: a clinical review. World Journal of Gastroenterology: WJG 2014;20(34):12144–60.
11. Younger DS. Treatment. In Human Lyme Neuroborreliosis. Chapter 10. Nova Biomedical: New York, 2015; 99.
12. Younger DS, Chen X. IVIg therapy in PANDAS: analysis of the current literature. J Neurol Neurosurg 2016;3(3):125.
13. Younger DS. Mold exposure and mycotoxicity: on the path to precise science. Blog. March 14, 2017; http://www.davidsyounger.com.
14. Hope J. A review of the mechanism of injury and treatment approaches for illness resulting from exposure to water-damaged buildings, mold, and mycotoxins. The Scientific World Journal 2013;2013:767482.
15. Younger DS. Water mercury toxicity: autoimmune insights for the brain. Blog. March 17, 2017; http://www.davidsyounger.com.
16. Younger DS. Autoimmune encephalitides. World Journal of Neuroscience 2017;7:327–61.
17. Beuker C, Schmidt A, Strunk D, et al. Primary angiitis of the central nervous system: diagnosis and treatment. Therapeutic Advances in Neurological Disorders 2018;11:1756286418785071.
18. Younger DS. Overview of primary and secondary vasculitides. In, The Vasculitides. Volume 1, David S. Younger, Ed. New York: Nova Science; 15–64.
19. Younger DS. Sports-related concussion in school-age children. World Journal of Neuroscience 2018;8:10–31.
20. Younger DS. Hashimoto's thyroiditis and encephalopathy. World Journal of Neuroscience 2017;7:307–26.
21. Wisniewski T, Goñi F. Immunotherapeutic approaches for Alzheimer's disease. Neuron 2015;85(6):1162–76.
22. Lee A, Gilbert RM. Epidemiology of Parkinson disease. Neurol Clin 2016;34:955–65.

BOX 6.1

COMMON SIDE EFFECTS OF IMMUNOTHERAPY PRESCRIPTION MEDICATIONS

Like any other medication, immunotherapy has risks and bene-fits. Virtually all potent immunosuppressants have the potential to overshoot their efficacy, and all have the potential to increase host susceptibility to infections. Corticosteroids in particular are known for the propensity to cause hypertension, hyperlipid-emia, hyperglycemia, peptic ulcer disease, moon face, and liver and kidney injury. The immunosuppressive drugs also interact with other medicines and affect their metabolism and action. Generally, many of the side effects can be averted by careful monitoring of blood tests.

Intravenous Immunoglobulin Therapy

IVIg is the most widely employed immune-modulating agent for autoim-mune neurological disorders. It is used in the treatment of post-infectious autoimmunity (I-Cubed) disorders where the immune system goes awry, leaving in its wake tandem central, peripheral, and autonomic nervous system dysfunction. Neurologists, rheumatologists, and immunologists presently have the most experience with IVIg therapies for serious autoimmune illness. However, it has always been a favored supplemental or replacement therapy for children with recurrent bacterial infections to restore immune function.

The idea behind IVIg is to usurp, or take control of, the immune response, especially at its final stage before complement is activated and there is irrevers-ible damage to parts of the nervous system targeted by the immune system. Proteins in the body act like the little bomb that says ACME in the old Road Runner cartoons. The Road Runner would invariably hand a bomb over to the coyote, at which point it would explode in his face. We can think of IVIg therapy as the thing that will defuse that bomb by dismantling the complement pathway like a bomb squad, but it also inhibits the secretion of cytokines. It is indicated therapy in children with IgG subclass deficiencies (usually involving IgG2 or IgG3), and in other disorders in which antibodies are within a normal quantitative range, but lack quality or the ability to respond to antigens as they normally should, resulting in an increased rate or increased severity of infections. In these situations, Ig infusions confer passive resistance to infection on their recipients by increasing the quantity/quality of IgG they possess.

This treatment can be administered through a home infusion agency that provides the drug and nursing personnel, or you can be treated in a doctor's office. Out-of-network home providers may be more expensive with considerable out-of-pocket expenditures than in-network specialty pharmacies and contracted nursing services. However, out-of-network providers will often accept insurance payments or negotiate rates, making them the superior choice for both the pharmaceutical and nursing services. There are a handful of highly recommended out-of-network providers in contrast to a cadre of in-network providers. With increasing trends for insurance carriers to package Ig products and nursing through national care managers, the onus falls more heavily on the treating neurologist to assure the highest level of available contracted care available from your insurance.

At a minimum, a patient receiving Ig therapy should be examined monthly, both at the outset of therapy to identify potential logistical and health-related issues, and to facilitate adjustments in the care plan. Afterward, arrangements made with the general practitioner or internist for regular follow-up visits at longer intervals will assure optimal therapy. The choice of a given regimen, administered weekly or over two consecutive days per month, is guided by the patient's tendency for side effects, which may include transient headache, fever, chills, rash, redness, flushing, nausea, myalgia, arthralgia, abdominal cramps, chest or back pain, and, rarely, aseptic meningitis or a severe allergic reactions.

Yet even before treatment begins, your physician will guide you through the arduous process of certification for IVIg treatment. The initial request for certification through a typical insurance plan usually triggers a sequence of reviews by insurance personnel that culminates in the final decision by a medical director, whose identity may not be readily apparent (you may be able to find them listed in your "determination of benefits letter" with the decision to cover treatment). In some instances, the insurance approval process drags on for weeks and even months, delaying the beginning of treatment unless the case is actively pursued by the ordering physician and home provider.

IVIg is a complex mixture drug comprising diverse human antibodies, all purified from the plasma of thousands of healthy donors. These treatments are highly valued because of their highly personalized nature, meeting the individual needs of each patient.[2] There are several product options to choose from. Approved IVIg products differ regarding source of plasma, isolation process, and formulation.

Your physician will choose the product that is right for you from among the available products. Brand names of IVIg products include:

- Gammagard
- Gamunex
- Octagam
- Privigen

A Typical IVIg Treatment Protocol

Therapy is generally administered for 3 to 6 months, and often longer until the desired effect is achieved. Before medication is administered, the patient is given intravenous saline to ensure hydration, as well as oral acetaminophen (Tylenol) and diphenhydramine (Benadryl) to treat and prevent allergic drug reactions. The administered dose is calculated by weight and administered via a slow drip, typically over 2 to 4 hours with frequent vital sign checks because both hypotension and hypertension may accompany an inadvertently fast infusion.

Subcutaneous (SC) Ig is an alternative preparation that is administered via a fine needle under the skin, much like insulin. In immunodeficiency the primary function of SC Ig is to replace missing antibodies. It is becoming increasingly popular among those who cannot tolerate intravenous injections due to migraine headache or other allergic reactions, and for those who require only a small dose. One benefit for some people is that it is self-administered and does not require a nurse. Brand names of subcutaneous formulations include HyQvia and Hizentra.[3]

PLASMA EXCHANGE

The last immune-modulatory therapy is plasma exchange, which filters your blood and removes, treats, and returns or exchanges blood plasma or components from and to the blood circulation. This process is used in the treatment for autoimmune disorders. It is rarely the primary therapy, instead used as adjunctive measure with other primary modalities. The usefulness of plasma exchange in treating autoimmune disorders is the ability to completely remove disease-causing autoantibodies from the circulation in the short-term, tempering the underlying disease process, while working alongside other immunosuppressive therapies for long-term benefit. Plasma exchange is frequently more expensive and less available than other immunotherapies because it is typically performed only in a hospital or affiliated outpatient unit, rarely in a physician's office. Though a plasma exchange is helpful in certain medical conditions, like any other therapy, there are potential risks and complications. Insertion of a rather large intravenous catheter can lead to bleeding, and, if the catheter is left in too long, it can cause infection.

Meet Cathy

My patient, Cathy, illustrates the complexity of treatment decisions where there are multiple triggers for brain dysfunction. I was only able to treat her effectively after a systematic evaluation and careful consideration of findings, which then led to creating a sensible treatment program tailored to her needs that was both safe and effective.

Cathy, a 16-year-old, was a normally functioning child, except for the fact that she had joint laxity, a connective tissue problem characterized by excessive flexibility of the ligaments and tendons, which was noted at age 6 by her dance teacher. Cathy also suffered from recurrent bouts of strep throat and fever, which was frequently treated with antibiotics beginning at age 3, and seemed to end following a tonsillectomy when she was 9. Yet that same year her mother found an engorged tick on her left ear that was not tested, nor was she tested or treated for Lyme disease. Following the tick incident, Cathy's mother noticed that Cathy began to suffer from involuntary movements of her arms and legs. She also complained of dizziness, unsteadiness, and anxiety. She had always been a strong math student, but by the time she was 10 she experienced difficulty in solving homework problems. She then reported headaches, memory loss, and reading difficulty.

By age 11, Cathy had difficulty walking down the hallways of her school. That was the last straw, and her mother took her to a Lyme specialist who tested Cathy, and she was found to be positive for Lyme and two other Lyme co-infections—*Babesia* and *Bartonella*. In recent years, we have found that these two additional infections are commonly carried by the same tick that is carrying Lyme disease. Cathy's treatment began with oral antibiotics that continued on and off for about 3 years; she returned to them whenever she experienced fevers.

Five years later, in February 2017, Cathy came to my office with weakness in the arms and legs and with difficulty walking, and she underwent neurophysiological testing that showed underlying peripheral demyelinating neuropathy of the legs and arm. She was lightheaded with attempted standing and found to have orthostatic hypotension with tilting upright and simultaneous measurement of heart rate and blood pressure, small fiber neuropathy on epidermal nerve fiber analysis of the calf and thigh, and a positive Lyme test. Her single photon emission computed tomography testing showed mild right temporal lobe hypoperfusion, and a positron emission tomography scan of the brain showed decreased metabolism in both temporal lobes and the cerebellum relative to the rest of the cerebral cortex. A low titer of the GAD65 antibody was found in her blood. This indicated a pervasive autoimmune process of the brain likely due to autoimmune encephalitis.

At this point we switched her medications completely. We started treating her with IVIg therapy, and within 6 months, her involuntary movements were reduced. By early 2018 she was still experiencing headaches, memory disturbances, fatigue, reading difficulties, and anxiety, and she was unable to attend school. The decision was made to continue IVIg and either start plasma exchange or biological therapy with Rituxan for presumptive autoimmune encephalopathy. After a single dose of rituximab, she noted marked symptomatic improvement in neurological complaints with improved gait, headaches, concentration, memory, and anxiety; however, reading difficulty persisted. However, for the first time Cathy was able to return to school, and she graduated high school with her classmates. A second treatment of Rituxan was given in the summer of 2018, and she has now been able to slowly taper down on the dose of IVIg and is completely off antibiotics.

MANAGEMENT OF NEUROPATHIC PAIN
WITH PRESCRIPTION MEDICATIONS

Small-fiber neuropathy (SFN)[4] is the best example of a nervous system disorder that is highly associated with pain and requires a systematic approach to pain management to alleviate the associated physical and mental anguish. SFN is a disorder of thinly myelinated (A-δ) and unmyelinated (C) fibers embedded in the skin. It is characterized by chronic and severe neuropathic pain, and occurs in association with various autoimmune disorders, such as metabolic (diabetes mellitus), infectious (Lyme disease), connective tissue disease (lupus and sarcoidosis), and genetic (Celiac disease). The incidence and prevalence of SFN is unknown, but an estimated 20 percent of patients with diabetes have painful neuropathy that is largely attributed to small-fiber involvement.

Non-steroidal anti-inflammatory drugs are useful anti-inflammatory agents for the "constitutional symptoms" of an autoimmune disorder such as low-grade aches and pains. However, they do not offer adequate analgesic relief for neuropathic pain associated with diabetes, Lyme disease, connective tissue disorders, Celiac disease, thyroiditis, and cancer. The pain associated with these autoimmune diseases can disturb an individual's quality of life.[4]

In 2017, researchers[5] found that disorders associated with pain ranked fifth among conditions cited by the Global Burden of Disease Study as a cause of years lived with disability.[6] Affected individuals cite, at best, modest clinically relevant benefit from any one intervention, suggesting the need for a multi-disciplinary approach to pain management.[7]

There are many prescription medications that can successfully manage this type of disabling pain. The first line of prescription medications for neuropathic pain are the gabapentinoids, notably Neurontin and Lyrica, which are also approved for the treatment of postherpetic neuralgia, which is neuropathic pain associated with diabetic neuropathy, fibromyalgia, generalized anxiety disorder, and restless leg syndrome. Some off-label uses of the gabapentinoids include the treatment of insomnia, migraine, social phobia, panic disorder, mania, bipolar disorder, and alcohol withdrawal.

Antidepressants are effective in the treatment of pain, but not all of them, and the ones that are effective do not all work to the same degree, or by the same mechanism. Tricyclic antidepressants are the most studied antidepressants for the treatment of neuropathic pain. They inhibit the reuptake of serotonin and norepinephrine at the synaptic level in the brain. Another group, the tertiary amines (e.g., amitriptyline [Elavil] and doxepin [Sinequan]), and imipramine (Tofranil) inhibit serotonin to a greater degree than norepinephrine. In contrast, the secondary amines (e.g., desipramine [Norpramin] and nortriptyline [Pamelor]) have more pronounced effects on norepinephrine. While these types of medications are reliable and effective, their use is often accompanied by weight gain and orthostatic hypotension, which in and of itself affects brain health.

Selective serotonin reuptake inhibitors (SSRIs) are another class of anti-depressants. To date, paroxetine (Paxil) and citalopram (Celexa) have demonstrated modest efficacy in the management of neuropathic pain, whereas fluoxetine (Prozac) has not demonstrated any efficacy at all. The overall impression is that SSRIs are less effective than other antidepressant options in the treatment of neuropathic pain. SSRI side effects also include weight gain and sexual dysfunction.

Selective serotonin norepinephrine reuptake inhibitors such as venlafaxine (Effexor) are yet another class of antidepressants. Despite a milder side effect profile than the tricyclic antidepressants, venlafaxine may elevate blood pressure, which can be very useful in patients with orthostatic hypotension. Bupropion (Wellbutrin) shows promise in managing pain, but is well known to lead to excessive appetite. Duloxetine (Cymbalta) is the only antidepressant approved by the US Food and Drug Administration for the treatment of neuropathic pain. It has been confirmed in several studies as an effective agent in the treatment of neuropathic pain. As for side effects, duloxetine may cause a host of brain health issues, including nausea, somnolence, dizziness, and fatigue.

Opioid analgesics (OxyContin, Oxycodone, Percocet), also referred to as "narcotics," are the most effective, but most often associated with addiction and the development of tolerance. Overuse or abuse of opioids have fueled what we now refer to as a very real opioid epidemic. Long-term opiate prescribing is also complicated by patients who divert or abuse their opioid analgesic medications. They have pharmacologic properties similar to those of morphine. This class of medication includes the derivatives hydrocodone, oxycodone, hydromorphone, codeine, and fentanyl and its analogs. They pass readily across nasal membranes as well as the BBB where they act at opiate mu receptor agonists leading to euphoria and analgesia.

Four historical developments have influenced the acceptance and availability of opioid analgesic drugs in the United States. First, the recognition of the appropriateness of opioid analgesic drugs for chronic pain treatment. Second, the recognition of a patient's right to pain relief by the medical professionals.[8] Third, the availability of opioid analgesic manufactured by the pharmaceutical industry, which aggressively markets addictive opioid analgesic drugs and the product Suboxone that combines buprenorphine with naloxone to treat opioid dependence.[9] Fourth, the establishment of guidelines by the Centers for Disease Control and Prevention (CDC) in 2016 for the safe dispensation of opioid analgesic drugs by community primary care providers and not just by pain management experts.[10] This was followed a year later by new evidence-based standards of the Joint Commission of the Accreditation of Healthcare Organization to improve the care of patients taking opioid analgesic drugs for chronic pain.[11]

In the search for alternatives, medical marijuana or "medical cannabis" has emerged as a likely favorite. Pharmaceutical grade cannabis derived from the *Cannabis sativa* plant employs tetrahydrocannabinol (THC) and other extractable plant compounds called phytocannabinoids or cannabinoids, such as cannabidiol (CBD), that act as agonists of the endocannabinoid system of receptors and neurotransmitters in the brain and immune system. Agonists of the endocannabinoid system regulate complex neurophysiological pathways involved in chronic pain[12] centered in frontal-limbic areas of the brain where the distribution of CB_1 receptors are most densely found,[13] whereas those affecting CB_2 receptors in the immune system attenuate low-grade inflammation.[14]

Other researchers[15] have more recently conducted a systematic review of randomized clinical trials of cannabis-based medications in the treatment of diverse autoimmune and non-autoimmune neurological disorders, and found cannabis-based medications to be effective. Cannabis-based medications showed a significant reduction in chronic pain compared to placebo in a cohort of over 1,300 patients, with a decrease in pain scores of two points in up to 50 percent of cases.[16] Finally, medical cannabis has the capacity to reduce opioid use while assuring a level of analgesia consistent with a quality of life, with significant cost savings[17] similar to patients who self-medicate with marijuana, and derive the same benefits of analgesia[18] due to the beneficial effects of cannabis.

Individuals seeking certification for a medical cannabis card in any of the US states with a dispensary program must see a physician who is enrolled in the program and can process their paperwork.

Meet Cindy

I first met Cindy more than 20 years ago when I was a young attending neurologist. Cindy had come in with numerous autoimmune disorders, beginning with myasthenia gravis (muscle weakness), lupus, and thyroiditis, as well as chronic inflammatory demyelinating polyneuropathy and postural orthostatic tachycardia syndrome. She had already been taking prednisone to treat her lupus for decades; however, she was unable to taper off of it. Worse, she developed the dreaded side effect of shingles, leading to post-herpetic neuralgia of the face as well as the associated painful blisters. IVIg gave her the option of tapering off of prednisone, as it controlled her auto-immune state, in an effort to avert further steroid side effects like diabetes, hypertension, and brittle bones.

Years later, Cindy was visiting me from Japan and Hong Kong where she had established residence with her husband. In Asia, she went back on prednisone and was prescribed opioids, and became addicted to OxyContin. After moving back to the United States two years ago, and unable to reduce her prednisone and opioids, I suggested adding medical cannabis to her IVIg, because of its purported analgesic benefits. Amazingly, she was able to taper off of both the prednisone and the opioids and has remained pain-free and in remission from all of her illnesses.

THE NEXT STEP

One of the best ways to maintain proper mental health is to follow the best practices of many effective types of therapy. In the next chapter, I will review a variety of complementary therapies that you can try right at home as the third step in the TAPES protocol.

7

Participate in Therapies that Address Stress and Mental Health Concerns

As you begin to identify your symptoms and address them with medication, it's very likely that your mental health issues will begin to resolve. Yet it's equally important to continuously pay attention to overt behavioral and affective symptoms and treat them as true health issues regardless of their cause.

Neuropsychiatric symptoms fall into two categories:

1. Behavioral symptoms are persistent or repetitive behaviors that are unusual, disruptive, inappropriate, or cause problems:

   - alterations in personal awareness, including neglect of hygiene and grooming
   - alterations in social awareness, lack of social tact, misdemeanors
   - early signs of disinhibition, sexual changes, violence, jocularity, restless pacing
   - mental rigidity and inflexibility
   - hyperorality: the compulsion to examine objects by mouth
   - stereotyped and perservative behavior
   - utilization behavior
   - distractibility, impulsivity, impersistence
   - loss of insight

2. Affective symptoms relate to mood:

- Depression
- Anxiety
- Sentimentality
- Suicidal and fixed ideation
- Delusion
- Hypochondriasis, bizarre somatic preoccupation
- Emotional unconcern, indifference, remoteness, apathy, lack of empathy and sympathy
- Inertia, spontaneity

Even with the best of health, we all have good days and bad days. Sometimes, the therapeutic approach is the best way to increase your resilience, so that you can bounce back from your bad days quickly and effortlessly.

This chapter is a guide to many useful therapeutic approaches. Some of them you can take on yourself, like meditation and mindfulness. However, some will require that you work with a licensed therapist. These trained and caring people can lend a hand in lightening your burden or provide guidance and assistance. Work with your current doctor to find the best therapists for you that practice these modalities.

CHOOSING THE RIGHT THERAPIST

There are many different types of mental health providers, and each has their own specialized training and expertise. There are social workers who understand social issues, and some of them may go on to develop expertise in psychology to psychoanalysis or talk therapy. There are clinical psychologists who delve more deeply into mental health and may have a more advanced understanding of brain function. Then there are psychiatrists, who are medical doctors and have learned the most important aspects of neurobiology and how it affects mental health, and how mental illness develops from various insults to the brain.

The most important shift in recent years is that the primary tool of psychiatrists has shifted from talk therapy to medication, because they understand that mental illness has a biological component. A psychiatrist is the only type of therapist that can prescribe medication, such as antidepressants, antipsychotics, anti-anxiety drugs (although any other medical doctor can do this as well). This is important because today we know that mental illness has a strong biological component that can be affected by insults in the course of neuro development, or due to genetic influences, or due to infectious and autoimmune insults throughout childhood and adulthood leading to disorders manifesting primary psychiatric symptoms—depression, anxiety, neuroses, etc. What's more, neurogenesis is not just restricted to early childhood: we now know that there are structures of the brain that can be influenced by medications, including the development of healthier synaptic connections that transfer information more quickly and more smoothly. In addition, those regions of the brain that are primarily concerned with mood and memory have been found to respond favorably to pharmacologic therapy.

In short, the right therapy can rewire the brain with lasting results. The best news is that you have choices: from the gentlest types of behavioral therapy to a medical response.

BOX 7.1

THE SECRET IS REGULATING STRESS

One of the key features of a healthy brain is resiliency: the ability to bounce back to a normal state after a traumatic event. Some of us seem more naturally resilient than others, and we used to believe that the secret to resiliency was adopting better mental health habits. However, new findings provide compelling evidence for the role that inflammatory and post-infectious autoimmune processes play in our ability to handle stress, including PTSD.[1] In fact, researchers have found that our ability to be resilient has more to do with biology than psychology.

Plasma and serum studies have found elevated levels of various inflammatory markers in PTSD patients compared to controls, and a recent meta-analysis of findings from 20 publications found the diagnosis to be reliably associated with elevated levels of circulating autoantibodies, including peripheral interleukin (IL)-6, IL-1β,

(Continued)

(*Box 7.1, continued*)

TNF-α, and interferon (INF)-γ.[2] Genetic studies link inflammation-related genes to risk for PTSD. What's more, studies showed that DNA methylation, the underlying mechanism of epigenetic regulation, is expressed differently depending upon the activity of inflammation and immune system genes.[3] This is big news for patients with PTSD, because it suggests that there may be an innate mechanism that determines an individual's ability to be resilient after a traumatic event, rather than blaming your symptoms on weak character.

MEDITATION

Meditation brings a state of profound, deep peace that occurs when the mind is calm and silent, yet completely alert. When we're anxious, we may feel disconnected from those around us. In order to heal, we need to learn how to take care of ourselves when we know we're upset or stressed. Meditation is one way that you can begin to focus on yourself so that you can heal, as you learn to put the outside world aside and create a space in which you can experience your feelings without reacting to them or being consumed by them.

Anyone can learn to meditate, regardless of religious affiliation or beliefs. In recent years, it has become more popular as we look for ways to unplug from technology and quiet our minds from our hectic lifestyles.

The science of meditation has seen huge growth over the last 30 years, and it is now thought to be one of the best-known tools for improving brain health on the physical, mental, and emotional planes. Research shows that an ongoing meditation practice can lead to increased development of several key areas of the brain, especially those related to higher-order cognitive functions. It has also been proven to increase brain activity and improve attention and concentration.[4] This benefit may be due to cognitive restructuring, autonomic changes, and the limited release of cytokines that occur during meditation. Recently, it has been shown that relaxation results in decreased levels of the antibodies IL-1 and IL-6. Therefore, reduction of cytokines by practicing meditation could well explain the enhanced cognition.

In the mental realm, meditation helps us learn how to be present, which enhances our attention skills by allowing us to let go of distractions and pay attention to only a few thoughts at a time. Emotionally, it allows us to let go of obsessive thoughts that can override our thinking brain, making them seem more real, scary, or more important than others. There is a growing body of evidence demonstrating positive benefits from meditation in stress reduction, anxiety, depression, and pain improvement. Its impact can be associated with the reversal of memory loss, reduction in anxiety, depression, and stress. Therefore, it is comforting to see that meditation can be considered in some instances an alternative medicine to conventional drug-centered therapies.

There has also been a tremendous increase in understanding the creativity process and how it enhances brain function,[5] especially in relation to meditation. A deep meditation practice and its associated relaxation techniques are thought to enhance access to creative cognition. Researchers suggest that meditation activates regions of the brain, particularly the frontal and parietal lobes, both of which are important for creative cognition. Meditation also impacts areas of the brain involved with autonomic nervous system function.

According to Bob Roth, the author of *Strength in Stillness: The Power of Transcendental Meditation*[6] and one of the best known meditation teachers, the common misconception about meditation is that all of its forms and techniques are practiced in the same way and produce roughly the same results. However, this is an overgeneralization. The mental procedures used by various traditions and schools of meditation can be very different. Recent scientific research has verified that these different ways of meditating activate different areas in our brain, culminating in different results.

Sam Katz, National Spokesman for Transcendental Meditation USA, sees meditation as common sense: just as weightlifting, tennis, and Pilates strengthen specific muscles and produce different overall effects in the body, so does focusing on a candlelight, repeating mantras, or trying dispassionately to observe one's mental content to induce changes in different areas of the brain. Three main meditation types can be recognized based on electroencephalographic (EEG) brain wave patterns that are produced. I discuss the results of each practice here below.

Type 1: Concentration or Focused Attention

Researchers have found that forms of meditation that involve a focus of attention (be it a physical object, a word, or a concept) increase the activity of beta (fast) EEG-waves that correspond to the active and attentive state of consciousness.

One study investigated a Tibetan Buddhist meditation technique, in which the attention was focused on "loving-kindness and compassion" towards other beings. Strong activity was found in brain areas responsible for processing sensory information, emotions and attention.

Type 2: Meditation of Observing the Mind: Open Monitoring

In several practices, like mindfulness meditation and some forms of Zen, no focus is present. Instead, the practitioner relies on an "open monitoring" of reality, during which one observes the contents of one's experience without judging them. There's no manipulation, just pure watchful presence. According to EEG-measurements, this contemplative sort of meditation increases the activity of slow theta waves, which reflects a relaxed state of mind.

Type 3: Meditation of Transcending: Automatic Self-Transcendence

According to scientific research, the practice of TM as taught by Maharishi Mahesh Yogi is unique in many a sense. Researchers created a separate, third category for this technique of automatic self-transcending, since the mental procedure transcends itself and culminates in a mental experience of "unboundedness."

The activity of the thalamus, the area responsible for processing sensory information, decreases with TM. On the other hand, the frontal areas of the brain, which are associated with higher executive functions and moral reasoning, become more active with TM. EEG recordings show that the activity of background alpha waves also increases, indicating relaxation and calm. What is even more interesting is that the overall coherence of brain waves increases during TM.

The overall huge growth and acceptance of TM in education, business, healthcare, and the general public has been due in large part to the extensive peer-reviewed research that has accumulated showing deep relaxation, reduction in stress and stress-related illness such as heart disease, and self-development aspects. TM is practiced for fifteen to twenty minutes twice per day and only taught by certified teachers through a standard course of instruction.

I am also an advocate of yoga and its meditative applications. Like TM, certain yoga techniques can shift mental activity into an enduring absence of narrative thought which improves the ability to focus and to spontaneously stay in the present moment.[7] This mental state of "thoughtless awareness" is associated with the experience of joy, a subsequent sense of relaxation and positive mood, as well as an increased understanding of the self. Studies have reported preliminary evidence of positive effects of yoga meditation in treating disorders such as asthma, epilepsy, ADHD, anxiety, and work stress.[8]

BOX 7.2

MEDITATION IS A PRACTICE

With certain meditation practices, in the beginning, you may feel slightly more agitated than relaxed. This happens because when you are quieting your mind, it might bring up negative or difficult emotions. However, with practice and the correct teacher, you will be able to acknowledge these thoughts, release them for the moment, and finally relax.

How to Meditate

Remember, you are not trying to get anywhere when you meditate. You are simply practicing the art of being here. You can meditate wherever you are most comfortable, sitting up or lying down. Wear comfortable, non-binding clothing, and find a quiet space where you won't be interrupted or distracted. Some people like to meditate in silence. Others enjoy listening to soft music, the sounds of nature or chanting, or following guided meditations that you can download. You might find it helpful to record yourself reading the following paragraph so that you can play it back during your practice (you can record it once, or several times in a row, depending on your preference). When you're ready to meditate, set aside as little as five minutes, and as you become more comfortable with the practice, it can last as long as you like, although rarely beyond twenty minutes.

Begin each meditation by closing your eyes and focusing attention on your mantra. Your breathing should be slow and rhythmic. After you close your eyes, notice when your attention is drawn to a thought, sound, sensation, or emotion. Simply allow yourself to have the experience without resisting it, and then gently bring your attention back to your breath. If you find yourself judging your thoughts as "wrong" or "bad," just notice the judgment as "thought," let it go, and bring your attention back to the breath.

Breathing for Meditation

Controlled, rhythmic breathing in and of itself is a type of relaxation therapy thought to reduce stress, increase alertness, and boost the immune system by activating the autonomic nervous system. Practiced for centuries by yogis, rhythmic and controlled breathing can play an important role in promoting in improving immunity and brain functioning. One theory of why it is so effective is that it regulates the ANS, which then sends a signal to the brain, causing a sense of calm, which controls the secretion of stress hormones like cortisol, epinephrine, and norepinephrine along the HPA axis. Controlled breathing also influences the immune system, reducing levels of cytokines at various intervals. When we're anxious or under stress, we inadvertently hold our breath or breathe much more shallowly. The key to breathing for meditation is to breathe more deeply and more consciously.

You can easily slow down your breathing by counting your breaths in your head. You can also experiment with breathing in through the nose and out through your mouth. This practice alone will automatically slow down your breathing.

The following exercise is a simple way for you to become more conscious of your breathing. You can use it any time, and especially during your meditation practice.

1. Sit upright and place your hands on your belly.
2. Slowly breathe in, expanding your abdomen for five counts as you breathe through the nose with your mouth closed.

3. Hold your breath for five counts.
4. Exhale through the nose or mouth for six counts.
5. Work your way up to repeating this pattern for 10 to 20 minutes a day for maximal gains.

MINDFULNESS

Mindfulness as a general concept and mindfulness meditation as a therapeutic method have become increasingly popular in the last decades.[9] Mindfulness-based stress reduction,[10] mindfulness-based cognitive therapy,[11] and other related interventions have proved effective in reducing stress, anxiety, and depression, and in improving general mental health and well-being.[12]

Mindfulness-based cognitive therapy can best be described in the words of its cofounder, John Teasdale,[13] who defines mindfulness as a mindful mode that is marked by "metacognitive awareness" or the deep, intuitive, experiential understanding (or insight) that thoughts and emotions are passing mental events, and not the reality of ones sense of self, the world, and the future. Teasdale contrasts the mindful "being mode" to the habitual "doing mode" which is marked by problem-solving and achievement-oriented thinking, both of which are characteristic of our everyday activities. When we practice mindfulness, we can let go of "rumination," a cognitive style marked by circular thinking about one's physical and emotional state. Rumination is considered part of the "doing mode" and is one of the traps we can fall into that can lead to a depressive state.[14]

Mindfulness meditation has been shown to significantly improve anxiety and pain. It is associated with heightened activation in regions involved in the cognitive and emotional evaluation of pain such as the orbitofrontal cortex, as well as decreased activation of sensory processing regions of the brain responsible for projecting the conscious experience of pain. The practice helps people shift their attention and engage with their breath; by doing so, they experience a decrease in pain.

As a mental practice, mindfulness teaches us how to pay more attention to whatever is going on around us. It allows you to focus on what you're choosing to be doing in the moment. When people cultivate mindfulness, their thinking becomes sharper. They're less distracted; they're less preoccupied with extraneous thoughts.[15] What's more, a mindfulness practice can improve memory, decrease stress, and increase overall happiness.[16]

How to Practice Mindfulness

A formal mindfulness practice is a structured experience like meditation, and the same instructions apply. Get comfortable and find a quiet space where you won't be interrupted or distracted. You might find it helpful to record yourself reading the following paragraph so that you can play it back during your practice (you can record it once, or several times in a row, depending on your preference). When you're ready to start this formal practice, set aside as little as 5 minutes, and as you become more comfortable with the practice, it can last as long as you like.

Begin by focusing attention on your breathing, which should be slow and rhythmic. Now, pay attention to what you are experiencing with your five senses (sight, hearing, tasting, touching, and smelling), your physical experience (how your body is feeling: heaviness, lightness, tension), your thoughts, and your emotions. Now, concentrate on just one of these experiences. This focal point could be your breath, a single object in front of you, or a sound. Your choice doesn't matter at all: the goal is to let your mind rest on just one stimulus. When you find your mind wander away from the focal point and other things come into your awareness, notice them, and then come back to your focal point. Gently let it go and come back to your breathing.

STAYING OPTIMISTIC WITH POSITIVE PSYCHOLOGY

Growing evidence has linked optimism and other positive psychological attributes to a lower risk of poor health outcomes.[17] One aspect of the famous Nurses' Health Study found that women in the highest quartile of optimism had the lowest risk for death from any cause including infection. Optimism has also been shown to be associated with a healthier lipid profile, lower levels of inflammatory markers, higher levels of serum antioxidants, and better immune responsiveness,[18] all of which are important for managing the symptoms of I-Cubed. In fact, staying optimistic is just as effective as many of the lifestyle behaviors discussed in this book, including following a healthy diet, engaging in physical activity, and achieving higher-quality sleep.[19]

Undue worrying and pessimism, like generalized anxiety disorder and depression, can be a common attribute for those suffering from autoimmune brain disorders. What's more, maintaining an optimistic outlook does not come easily. Our disposition can be a result of both nature (our genetics) and nurture (our environment, including the attitudes of our parents). However,

BOX 7.3

TECHNOLOGY TO THE RESCUE

There are exciting new technological tools, referred to as eHealth options, that have been proven to reduce and manage stress, reduce depression, track sleep, and teach impulse control for those with obsessive compulsive disorder. Scientific studies focusing on eHealth has grown rapidly over recent years with several controlled trials in the field of anxiety disorders, mood disorders, and behavioral medicine. Two meta-analyses found that eHealth interventions could both reduce and prevent depression and anxiety.[20,21]

As you'll learn in chapter 8, physical activity is key component to maintaining and improving mental health. Technology can help us track our exercise time and movements into quantifiable outputs through devices like Fitbits. These activity trackers can provide feedback and offer interactive behavior change tools that are motivating, helping users reach daily or longer-term goals, such as counting steps taken throughout the day.

working on becoming more optimistic is under our control. There is no easy antidote to spiraling worries, but formulating concrete plans and actions that keep you focused on the daily pace of your life, as well as the behavioral modifications discussed in this chapter, are good remedies.

PETS BOOST MENTAL HEALTH

It is well known that pets can have a profound effect on the psychological state of their owners, offering reassurance, friendship, and compassion. According to new research,[22] companion animals improve mental and emotional well-being, as pet owners are less likely to suffer from stress, anxiety, and depression than people without pets. Pet therapy improves a wide array of mental health disabilities, including anxiety, panic, post-traumatic stress, mood obsessive compulsive, and other disorders. What's more, dog owners who walk their dogs are significantly more likely to be physically active, which in and of itself improves mental health.

The well-documented effects include increased social attention, increased social behavior, increased interpersonal interactions, and reduced depression while increasing mood. People with pets overall experience a decrease in fear and anxiety and a promotion of calmness. There is also some evidence for positive effects on the immune system overall, a reduction in aggression, and enhanced empathy and improved learning. In a 2012 study, researchers found that pets activate the oxytocinergic system through social interaction between people and pets. This relationship may also lead to reduced cortisol levels, both of which are biological functions of managing stress.[23]

It seems that any pet will do the job. However, specifically trained service dogs and other emotional support animals (ESAs) are a little known yet highly effective treatment for mental illness. ESAs are typically dogs, but can be cats or other animals. The animal does not have to receive specialized training to become an ESA. A trained psychiatric service dog can be the difference between being free to interact and enjoy life, or being limited by isolation and fear.

As defined in the Americans with Disabilities Act, a service dog is "trained to do work or perform tasks for the benefit of an individual with a disability, including a physical, sensory, psychiatric, intellectual, or other mental disability." A psychiatric service dog is further defined as one trained to "detect the onset of psychiatric episodes, and lessen their effects." These canines undergo vigorous training to earn their title. Dogs can be trained to recognize seizures, hypoglycemia, and post-traumatic stress and anxiety disorders. They are trained to track movement and sense anxiety.

Children interact with dogs in other ways that may benefit them. Pet therapy affects children's mental health and developmental disorders by reducing anxiety and arousal or enhancing attachment. In fact, children often rank pets higher than humans as providers of comfort and self-esteem and as confidants.[24] A pet can stimulate conversation for children, acting as an icebreaker that can alleviate social anxiety. Companionship with a pet can also reduce separation anxiety and strengthen attachment.

Service dogs may help improve well-being, self-esteem, and an individual's psychosocial situation.[25] These dogs perform tasks to mitigate the problem and calm the handler. They can stop self-harm behavior by barking and calling attention to others, and nudging their noses between the person's hands.

COGNITIVE BEHAVIORAL THERAPY

One particularly effective and often used therapy to treat a range of neuropsychiatric disorders, from anxiety and OCD to depression, is cognitive behavioral therapy (CBT). This problem-focused and action-oriented mode differs from historical approaches to psychotherapy, such as psychoanalysis, where the therapist looks for the unconscious meaning behind the behaviors and then formulates a diagnosis.

The premise of CBT is that our moods are created by our thoughts. This belief plays out in the following assumptions:

1. You feel the way you do right now because of the thoughts you are thinking.
2. When you are feeling depressed your thoughts are dominated by pervasive negativity.
3. Negative thoughts contain gross distortions.

Individuals with impaired thought processing will have self-esteem issues, which magnifies trivial mistakes or imperfections into an overwhelming feeling of personal defeat. Overcoming a sense of worthlessness is accomplished by targeting these same negative thoughts, writing each of them down, and equating them to a list of ten specific cognitive distortions. By substituting a rationale statement for the negative thought, it is possible to recognize self-defeating thoughts as they arise, understand them, and the talk back to them, disarming the internal critic that dwells in your mind.

Patients report that through a combination of CBT therapy and proper medication, their depression lifts, and they can have a transcending experience. Coupled with active psychiatric care, the great contribution of CBT has been the circumvention of long and often painstaking psychoanalysis that takes years. In addition, possibly equally important, most health insurance companies cover this type of therapy.

There are many books available that address CBT in detail, and *Feeling Good, The New Mood Therapy*, by Dr. David Burns, is an excellent resource.[26] Burns was a student of Dr. Aaron Beck, who is credited with originating CBT to treat depression.[27] Beck, at some point in his career as a psychiatrist, lost confidence in psychoanalysis in the most disturbed patients. He devised a program called *mental health hygiene*, which is how a patient presents to the world. His therapeutical model helps individuals unravel their thought constructs, so that they can see that they are thinking in a disturbed fashion. He found, as many CBT therapists now do, that when people can understand their false thinking, they wake up and can change, without spending years in psychotherapy.

ACCEPTANCE AND COMMITMENT THERAPY

Acceptance and commitment therapy (ACT) is a psychological treatment with a clear theoretical basis. The underlying theory is that psychological problems develop through the inappropriate or unhelpful regulation of behavior inflexibility in relation to environmental contingencies.[28] Rather than changing your beliefs, ACT aims to reduce the extent to which the same beliefs and other symptoms dominate your conscious experience and behavior. More specifically, treatment of symptoms is not focused on their removal, but on taking them less literally and disrupting their link with behavior.

At its core, ACT is a behavioral treatment grounded in producing functional change. As the name suggests, ACT has two broad components. In the acceptance component, therapists help the individual recognize and dispassionately observe symptoms and their associated reactions. The commitment component emphasizes one's personal values and goals, and seeks to minimize the effects of symptoms on achieving those goals in behavioral terms. Diffusion techniques are particularly effective in reducing repetitive cognitive processes such as depressive rumination, anxious worry, and persistence of obsessive thoughts.

ACT therapists use experiential exercises, illustrative metaphors, and behavioral tasks in order to effect change, with logical analysis having a relatively minor role. Although ACT is often described as a variant of CBT, the overlap in therapeutic elements is small.

Two randomized clinical trials tested the application of ACT on patients suffering from acute psychosis with surprisingly powerful outcomes. Bach and Hayes[29] assessed the impact of ACT on patients with psychotic symptoms and found that their mental health improved at twice the rate of patients following a CBT approach.

A popular book published in 2010, *Things Might Go Terribly, Horribly Wrong: A Guide to Life Liberated from Anxiety*, by Kelly Wilson,[30] reviews ACT for lay readers. You can also work with your physician to find a therapist trained in ACT techniques.

DIALECTICAL BEHAVIORAL THERAPY

Among the psychosocial treatments showing efficacy for bipolar disease, dialectical behavior therapy (DBT), a comprehensive cognitive behavioral treatment, has gained the most empirical support. It involves weekly hour-long individual therapy, weekly group skills training, and between-session telephone consultation to coach the patient in the use of behavioral skills, and weekly therapist consultation team meetings designed to support, motivate, and enhance the skills of therapists.[31] However, standard DBT is lengthy and resource intensive: it typically takes a full year to go through this therapeutic process.

COMBATTING ADDICTION

With approximately 41 percent of 18- to 24-year-olds enrolled in a degree-granting institution after high school,[32] college students, especially those at residential colleges,[33] are at heightened risk of drinking heavily with a myriad of associated negative consequences. This includes blackout attacks, unplanned sexual activity, social and interpersonal problems, and frank alcohol abuse and dependence. The latter can be an especially worrisome outcome in college students exposed to hazing when rushing a fraternity or sorority. Typically designed to establish or confirm group loyalty, hazing employs alcohol consumption, as well as, illilcit drug use, humiliation, isolation, sleep-deprivation, and sex acts. Students who successfully complete the program become the future generation of hazers perpetuating the cycle, while those who do not succeed are fortunately spared the cycle of doing it to others. Almost all of the acts that they engage in would constitute misconduct by the school if found out, however such practices tend to be secretly condoned by generations of fraternity or sorority alumni, and are often ignored by university officials until a catastrophe occurs. There is a large gap between the number of students who report experience with hazing behaviors and those that label their experience as hazing. The tough road to recovery is when a student becomes an alcoholic because of fraternity behavior, as such students often experience later school or career disruptions and failures.

The twelve steps to recovery, listed in the so-called Big Book or bible entitled *Alcoholics Anonymous*[34] and advocated by AA groups, have been a resource for generations. First published in 1939, the organization's success is based upon relating stories of inspiration and recovery. Groups meet every day in every city across the country, and on every college campus, to encourage sobriety at all ages, and to reduce the emotional and physical impact of alcohol on the body and especially the nervous system.

Meet Sam

A 20-year-old college sophomore was rushing a fraternity at a well-known university that included compulsory drinking of large quantities of alcohol for several weeks, as well as use of a variety of illicit substances including recreational cocaine. Oblivious to its impact, his parents helped him complete the semester and then brought him back home for the summer. When at home, it was apparent that his behavior had changed, and he had developed an addiction to alcohol and illicit drugs. He had a history of a concussion complicated by mood disturbances, and was gluten-free because of Celiac disease. He also had a mildly reduced IgG and IgA subclass levels in a prior routine blood test. He had gone off his diet during the period of hazing and was eating lots of fast-food and even started smoking cigarettes to look cool. Sam voluntarily admitted himself, with the support of his family, to a psychiatric unit for college students with similar problems to safely withdraw from alcohol and drugs. He was placed on naltrexone 50 mg to reduce his urge to drink and drug cravings, and transferred to an inpatient substance use rehabilitation program using extensive DBT, and Alcoholics Anonymous (AA) group meetings. Two weeks later he was successfully detoxed and released to a day program, which he continued until starting college in the fall. In the meantime, he received a small monthly dose of intravenous immune globulin (IVIg) to stabilize his immune system.

8

Eat and Exercise to Restore Brain Health and Reset the Immune System

As you've learned, lowering inflammation is a primary goal for anyone suffering from an autoimmune disease, and it is even more critical for someone suffering with brain health symptoms. Systemic inflammation accompanies a variety of allergic, autoimmune, infectious, toxic, and metabolic brain processes, traumatic brain injury, and neurological hereditary disorders. Even low-grade inflammation promotes disturbance of the BBB. When this occurs, brain cells secrete inflammatory molecules, called cytokines, which disturb normal functioning and can lead to a range of cognitive and neuropsychiatric manifestations.

Preempting this process would have been unthinkable until recently. Researchers have discovered startling new and effective ways to promote brain health through anti-inflammatory protocols, much like my TAPES program. We now know that by reducing inflammation throughout the brain and the body, you may be able to reset your immune system without medication and at the same time enhance many different cognitive functions, feel calmer, and sleep better.

Luckily, one of the easiest ways to lower inflammation is with lifestyle changes, like following the right diet and exercising regularly. These suggestions turn out to be sound medical advice for a myriad of reasons that you'll learn about in this chapter. But perhaps the most important is paying attention to one's epigenetics for they are often the key factors for silencing one's genetic predisposition for not only illness, but also the activation of infections and inflammation.

Recent findings[1] show that the onset and development of mental illnesses cannot be described by a one-gene/one-disease approach. Instead, they are thought to result from the interplay of a large number of genes, each of which can be affected by our environment, creating the epigenetic changes that influence our ability to turn on and off these genes. Environmental factors such as diet and infections can play a significant role in these epigenetic modifications, and ultimately influence neuropsychiatric disorders.

HYDRATION SUPPORTS BRAIN HEALTH

You might be surprised to learn that staying properly hydrated is one of the best ways to support your body's metabolism and immune system, and it's crucial to brain health. The majority of your body's mass is comprised of water, ranging from 75 percent in infants to 55 percent in the elderly. And because of this, we know that every bodily process, and every living cell, depends on water to function properly.

Although it is well known that water is essential for our survival, only recently have we begun to understand its role in the maintenance of brain function. Current findings in the field suggest that particular cognitive abilities and mood states are positively influenced by water consumption. The impact of dehydration on cognition and mood is particularly relevant for those with poor fluid regulation, such as the elderly and children.

Nutritional and physiological research teams have described the daily total water intakes of children, women, and men, yet there is no widespread consensus regarding the how much water each of these different demographic groups requires. Dehydration, or even inadequate hydration, meaning a loss of only 1 to 2 percent of body water, can be the singular cause of a wide variety of brain health symptoms, including impaired cognitive performance, fatigue, mood shifts, muddled thinking, inattentiveness, and poor memory. We lose water every day through the skin, lungs, kidneys, and digestive tract—in other words, by sweating, breathing, and the elimination of waste. Checking the color of your urine can be a useful indicator of adequate hydration; it should be almost colorless, with a brighter color signaling dehydration.

Determining how much water you need to drink or get from the foods you eat is an entirely personal equation. You need to factor in your age, activity level, environmental conditions, and whether you ingest water in foods already in your diet like fresh fruits and vegetables. More than two dozen fruits and vegetables are especially hydrating, including:

- Apples
- Bananas
- Blueberries
- Broccoli

- Carrots
- Cauliflower
- Cucumbers
- Grapes

- Lettuce
- Pears
- Peppers
- Pineapple

- Spinach
- Strawberries
- Tomatoes
- Watermelon

THE BEST FOODS FOR BRAIN HEALTH

It is becoming increasingly clear that the best diet for both the brain and the immune system is one and the same: an anti-inflammatory one. I support a hybrid version of two popular diets: The Mediterranean Diet and the Dietary Approaches to Stop Hypertension (DASH) diet, together called the Mediterranean-DASH Intervention for Neurodegenerative Delay, or MIND. This eating plan was developed based on exhaustive research and identifies the nutrients, foods, and dietary patterns related to improving brain health.

The MIND diet was first introduced in 2015. Its primary goal is to reduce both inflammation as well as oxidative stress in the brain and body,[2] and early studies have demonstrated its success. Oxidative stress occurs when unstable molecules called *free radicals* accumulate in large quantities, they damage our cells, causing particularly devastating results in the brain. The foods featured in the MIND diet are high in antioxidants, which are known to combat inflammation and protect the brain from oxidative stress.[3] One observational study found that people who followed the MIND diet the closest experienced a slower decline in brain function.[4]

The MIND diet emphasizes natural plant-based foods, particularly berries and green leafy vegetables, which has been associated with a slower rate of cognitive decline, a better protection against overall aging as well as dementia.[5,6] It also includes limited amounts of animal proteins, white-colored seafood, tasteful high-fiber sources, smart carbohydrates, healthy fats, and calcium-rich foods.

The following are the top ten foods the MIND diet encourages.[7] The path to linking optimal brain health with making good food choices can begin as early as childhood, by setting family rules surrounding strong food habits and sensible nutrition. The MIND diet guidelines are appropriate for the entire family. My suggestion is to make sure you and your family eats at least one of the following foods at every meal:

- Green, leafy vegetables: kale, spinach, cooked greens, and salads.
- All other vegetables: Choose non-starchy vegetables because they have lots of nutrients with fewer calories.
- Berries: strawberries, blueberries, raspberries, and blackberries are all packed with antioxidants.
- Nuts: A variety of nuts will allow you to obtain a variety of nutrients.
- Olive oil: Use olive oil as your main cooking oil for sautéing. Fried foods are prohibited on this diet.
- Whole grains: oatmeal, quinoa, brown rice, whole-wheat pasta, and 100 percent whole-wheat bread.
- Fish: Choose fatty fish like salmon, sardines, trout, tuna, and mackerel for their omega-3 fatty acids.
- Beans: all beans, lentils, and soybeans.
- Poultry and lean meats: occasionally, and never the predominant food on your plate.
- Wine: Both red and white wine may benefit the brain. Limit to a glass a day.

HEALTHY FATS OPTIMIZE BRAIN HEALTH

For decades, dietary guidelines have focused on reducing total fat and saturated fatty acid intake, based on the presumption that replacing saturated fatty acids with carbohydrates and unsaturated fats will lower low-density lipoprotein cholesterol and reduce cardiovascular and cerebrovascular disease. This focus was largely based on some observational and clinical data, despite the existence of several randomized trials and observational studies that did not support these conclusions.[8]

Today, we feel very differently about eating healthy fats, and some of my recommendations may seem counterintuitive. New research[9] emphasizes the importance that fats or "lipids" play in the structural and functional role of maintaining healthy neurons and preserving brain health. Lipids can affect multiple brain processes by regulating synaptic transmission, membrane fluidity, and signal-transduction pathways. This means that a diet high in healthy fats improves your thinking speed as well as the integrity of your blood–brain barrier, which is especially critical for thwarting autoimmune processes.

Foods contain a mixture of different types of fats, including saturated fatty acids or polyunsaturated fatty acids (PUFAs), depending on their chemical structure. Their impact on your health strongly depends on the types of fat you eat, as well as the quantity. Omega-6 and omega-3 PUFAs are the most nutrient-dense and have the greatest anti-inflammatory potential.[10] During the initial phase of an inflammatory response, PUFA metabolism switches to the production of lipoxins, which can limit the extent and duration of the inflammatory process and promote an early resolution. Diets with low levels of PUFA and omega-6 and omega-3 are associated with neuropsychiatric and neurological disorders with inflammatory outcomes, whereas dietary omega-3 PUFAs support cognitive processes and maintain synaptic functions and plasticity.[11] Diets that are high in saturated fats negatively affect brain functions and increase the risk of neurological diseases.[12] What's more, shifting away from a diet high in processed carbohydrates to incorporate more heathy fats may also help improve insulin levels and reduce the risk of diabetes, which is one of many endocrine disorders that affect thinking.

One easy change we can all make is switching back to whole milk and whole milk products, unless of course you are lactose intolerant. Whole milk contains the healthy fatty acids and is now thought to provide better nutrition, weight management, and immune competence as compared to skim milk or reduced fat milk. For instance, one cup of whole milk per day leads to vitamin D levels comparable to that of adolescents who ingested up to three cups of 1 percent milk, and is also associated with a likelier lean body mass. It also turns out that a handful of nuts a day, which are packed with healthy fats, reduces the risk of infectious illnesses that can cause brain health problems.

THE IMPORTANCE OF PROTEINS

You also need to incorporate lots of healthy protein sources into your meals. These can be vegetarian options like beans and grains, yet I do not advocate for a strict vegan diet, one devoid of all foods from animals: the proteins in plants are not considered to be "complete" and must be balanced by consuming complementary sources. Though most Americans rely too heavily on animal foods for protein, getting quality protein from dairy, like yogurts, and eggs can round out your options.

Fish is another great suggestion for high-quality protein that also offers a nutritious bonus of omega-3 fatty acids, and particularly PUFAs. Eating fish has been repeatedly shown to foster optimal brain development. Omega-3 PUFAs offer neuroprotective properties.[13] There are two distinct types: DHA stands for *docosahexaenoic acid* and EPA stands for *eicosapentaenoic acid*.

DHA is quantitatively the most important omega-3 PUFA in the brain, and its role has just recently been explored in adult neurogenesis.[14] Beneficial effects in mood disorders have been reported in clinical trials featuring fish oils high in EPA; other neurodegenerative conditions such as Alzheimer's disease have been studied in relationship to DHA supplementation.

Some of the best fish choices are fatty cold-water fish, because they are high in omega-3 fatty acids. These include:

- Black cod
- Bluefish
- Herring
- Mackerel
- Salmon
- Sardines

SHOULD I TRY GOING GLUTEN OR SUGAR-FREE?

Gluten-free and sugar-free diets are all the rage, and there may be a good reason why. Your brain health symptoms might be directly related to the foods you choose to eat. I suggest to all of my patients that they try a modified elimination diet, and stop eating gluten and sugar completely for at least two weeks to see if their cognitive issues reverse. If you don't feel better at all after two weeks, you'll know that these foods are not a problem.

Sugar has been used in meal preparation for over 10,000 years.[15] By 1800, the average American consumed approximately seven pounds of sugar a year.[16] Today, we consume over 100 pounds of added sugar annually,[17] and according to the CDC[18] more than one in four persons in the United States has a disease related to eating too much sugar. Categorized as metabolic syndrome, these diseases include hypertension, dyslipidemia, type 2 diabetes, obesity, and cardiovascular complications.[19] Sugar glycates, or coats, red and white blood cells and other immune cells that are responsible for the immune response, altering their function and increasing inflammation.

Our craving for sugar is likely rooted in our brain circuits dedicated to reward the recognition of high-energy food sources, which was critical for our survival.[20] However, these numbers, and the well-documented incidence of obesity related to excessive sugar consumption, suggest that we are eating much more sugar than we need. Removing added sugars from your diet is one of the easiest ways to boost your own immune response. My patients also find that by consuming less sugar, especially in the evenings, they sleep better at night and think more clearly during the day.

Gluten sensitivity found in Celiac disease is a real problem because the disease it causes exists on a spectrum from mild gastrointestinal symptoms to full-blown induced systemic and nervous system autoimmunity. For more information about Celiac disease and gluten sensitivity, see chapter 12.

LEPTIN AND THE NEURAL BASIS OF HUNGER

Many doctors now will measure leptin levels in both overweight and anorexic individuals as a quantifiable way to determine brain health. Leptin is a hormone that innately controls hunger and satiety. Low levels of circulating leptin prevent the brain for registering when you are feeling full after a meal and can be a cause of overeating and obesity. Normal circulating levels are related to satiety, and high levels signal the brain that you are full all the time, regardless of whether you have eaten.

Leptin has a secondary role as a cytokine and promotes inflammatory responses. Elevated levels of circulating leptin in obese patients contribute significantly to the low-grade inflammatory state that makes those individuals more susceptible to develop cardiovascular diseases, type II diabetes, or degenerative disease, in addition to autoimmune disease. Conversely, reduced levels of leptin such as those found in malnourished individuals have been linked to increased risk of infection and reduced cell-mediated immunity. Leptin also has fundamental roles in glucose and lipid homeostasis, reproduction, immunity, inflammation, bone physiology, and tissue remodeling.

BOX 8.1

CHANGE THE WAY YOU THINK ABOUT DIETING

The path to optimal brain health begins in childhood with good food habits and sensible nutrition. For adults, optimal brain and body health can only truly be assured by achieving one's ideal weight. Psychologist and diet expert Dr. Stephen Gullo, author of *The Thin Commandments Diet*,[21] notes that caloric intake is only half the success story, the other half being able to uncover the individual's unique daily eating. With the right strategy, you can expect to shift from being a dieter to a food strategist in implementing a way of eating that avoids harmful weight fluctuations.

THE STORY BEHIND *THE WAHLS PROTOCOL*

It is becoming clear that anti-inflammatory regimens benefit people with autoimmune diseases with the most successful ones being those that encompass lifestyle changes. One such multifaceted and holistic approach came from the personal experience of Dr. Terry Wahls, who developed progressive multiple sclerosis (MS), a disease that slowly advances toward a wheelchair. Her personal odyssey of how she happened upon an all-encompassing protocol through self-reflection and uncontrolled patient observational studies of similarly affected cases of MS was first published in the *Journal of Alternative and Complementary Medicine* in 2014.[22]

Wahls, who practiced dance and Tae Kwon Do, and suffered loss of stamina and strength, was put off by traditional medicine when her illness struck. Growing steadily weaker, and losing more and more function and activity tolerance, she became bedridden and was at a crossroads despite conventional medicine. She believed she had only two options: accept her disability despite optimal medical treatment for MS, or increased involvement in her healthcare. She chose the latter.

Translating animal research of mouse doses to human ones, she first added B vitamins, omega-3 fatty acids, alpha lipoic acid, coenzyme Q, and L-carnitine to her daily diet, and saw a slowing of her own illness. She added electrostimulation and started an aggressive program of physical therapy and daily exercise. She recognized the importance of micronutrients including sulfur amino acids, iodine, flavonoids, and vitamin D in her daily regimen for optimal brain health. Later she incorporated dietary foods that contained vitamins, minerals, and essential fatty acids.

Her new diet translated into nine cups of vegetables and fruit each day, with grass-fed meat and wild fish. Determined to optimize everything, she looked more deeply at the environmental factors associated with poorly explained neurological and psychological symptoms. Two stood out: food allergies and toxic load. Her interpretation of the scientific literature suggested that food sensitivities or allergies were a likely cause for a number of neurological and psychological symptoms. She prophylactically eliminated the most common offenders of gastrointestinal intolerance, namely, gluten, dairy, and eggs. She also incorporated her insights into the lowering the body's toxic load, reducing her exposure to mercury (frequently found in fish), herbicides, and pesticides (by eating organic foods), and by improving the ability to excrete toxins by adding methylated folate, B12, sulfur amino acids, and fiber to her dietary regimen.

Two months after starting electrostimulation therapy, exercise, and intensive nutrition, Dr. Wahls was able to sit in a standard desk chair without being exhausted and later reclaimed the ability to walk, and then run, and ultimately ride a bicycle.

BOX 8.2

DIETS BOOKS TO CONSIDER

"The road to recovery starts with taking personal charge, acting like a detective, being on the lookout for brain dysfunction resulting from gluten sensitivity, excessive carbohydrate and dietary sugar ingestion." So states neurologist Dr. David Perlmutter, author of *Grain Brain* and *The Better Brain Book*.[23] Shifting your focus from carbohydrates to heathy fats is his main recommendation. Perlmutter believes, as I do, that a diet incorporating healthy fatty acids and monosaturated fats reduces inflammation. The antioxidant action of dietary cholesterol, found in foods like eggs, protects the brain from the damaging effects of free radicals.

The Autoimmune Fix,[24] developed by the functional medicine practitioner Dr. Tom O'Bryan, seeks to stop hidden autoimmune damage through his two-phase dietary protocol. He is a strong advocate for removing gluten, sugar, and even dairy to lower inflammation and prevent the autoimmune response from recurring. A 3-week elimination-style diet completely removes gluten, dairy, and sugar. One can eat all forms of seasonal fruits, vegetables, and nuts; non-factory farm-raised meats and fish; and fermented foods. The second phase eliminates other typical offenders that can trigger allergies or food sensitivities, along with other immune-mediated symptoms. In this phase he removes soy; all remaining grains such as corn, rice, and quinoa; nightshade vegetables; and FODMAP fresh and dried fruits, nuts and seeds, and vegetables, which you'll learn more about in chapter 12.

(Continued)

(*Box 8.2, continued*)

Lastly, optimal brain health is related to maintaining one's ideal weight. Psychologist and diet expert Dr. Stephen Gullo, author of *The Thin Commandments Diet*, has developed an eating plan that follows many of the same guidelines I've outlined in this chapter. It's also full of tasty recipes that make losing weight less of a chore, because the foods he promotes focus on increasing your body's metabolism without portion restriction.

THE IMPORTANCE OF EXERCISE FOR BRAIN HEALTH

Exercise can be very beneficial for those with neurological disturbances, because exercise enhances brain health in many different ways. It facilitates neural plasticity through the availability of specific proteins in the brain and muscles of the body, such as brain-derived neurotrophic factor (BDNF), which aids in the growth of new neurons as well as the survival and function of existing brain cells. New research shows that the hippocampus, the part of the brain that aids in spatial navigation and memory formation, is substantially affected by physical activity.

If you are suffering from symptoms related to attention, spatial memory, working memory, and even processing speed, studies have shown clear improvements with exercise[25] in adults and children, including increases in academic achievement. For instance, exercise helps the brain by making it more receptive to new information. Lui and investigators[26] constructed a study with the aim of testing the influence of physical activity on learning a second language and demonstrated that foreign speakers with only a basic knowledge of English benefited from physical activity in learning new sets of words. Exercise is also an important environmental factor that can lower the risk for various complex diseases including those that affect the brain, including Parkinson's disease and dementia. What's more, both epidemiological and intervention studies indicate that exercise may delay or prevent the onset of Alzheimer's disease.[27]

According to a review of research regarding the link between mood and physical activity, people who work out even once a week or for as little as 10 minutes a day tend to be more cheerful than those who never exercise. A number of studies have noted that physically active people have much lower risks of developing depression and anxiety than people who rarely move. A review of 49 prospective studies[28] examining over 250,000 subjects found that those who exercised regularly had overall lower odds of developing depression. This finding was even more pronounced in children, suggesting that there is a protective effect of exercise.

In all of these studies, the type of exercise did not seem to matter. Some happy people walked or jogged. Others practiced yoga-style posing and stretching. In addition, the amount of exercise needed to influence happiness was slight. Several studies included subjects who worked out only once or twice a week, and reported that they felt happier than those who never exercised. In other studies, 10 minutes a day of physical activity was linked with buoyant moods.

However, more movement generally contributes to greater happiness. In one study, those who exercised for at least 30 minutes on most days, which is the current US and European standard recommendation for good health, were 30 percent more likely to consider themselves happy than people who did not meet the guidelines. The latest research shows that exercise not only affects and modulates depression—it can prevent it. A 2018 study published in the *Journal of the American Medical Association* found that higher levels of physical activity were linked to reduced odds for major depression.[29]

Yet keep in mind that physical activity can be a double-edge sword. I cannot stress enough the importance of taking on an exercise program that is well supervised and within your current health status: don't take on too much too soon. In the absence of a well-constructed and supervised program, you may be putting yourself at risk for a concussion. Among 3,427 children who were physically active for an hour per day 5 days per week or more playing a team sport, 20 percent reported a sports-related concussion in the preceding 12 months.[30]

LIMITED MOVEMENT MIGHT BE AFFECTING YOUR BRAIN HEALTH

Exercise can benefit overweight individuals, and recent research suggests that some types of exercise may be better than others. The arithmetic involved seems straightforward: exercise burns calories during exercise and, over time, should drop pounds. However, the reality is more complex because most people who start exercising lose fewer pounds than would be expected, given the number of calories they are burning during workouts. Some even gain weight. According to a 2017 study,[31] vigorous running halted acylated ghrelin production, a hormone associated with hunger, more than gentler jogging. So whenever possible, increase the length and intensity of your workouts for the greatest weight loss benefits.

Sitting for hours at a time slows cerebral blood flow (CBF), a recognition that has implications for long-term brain health. Decreased CBF is associated with lower cognitive functioning and increased risk of neurodegenerative diseases, because prolonged sitting impairs peripheral blood flow and function. A study published in the *Journal of Applied Physiology*[32] explored the effect of uninterrupted sitting and found that prolonged, uninterrupted sitting in healthy desk workers reduced CBF; however, this effect was offset when frequent, short-duration walking breaks were incorporated. Getting up from your desk for just 2 minutes every half-hour may prevent a decline in CBF and may even increase it. Consider setting your computer or phone to beep every half-hour. Then, when it goes off, get up and take a short walk around your office or home.

Some people worry that they are too old to exercise, or that they missed the boat and won't be able to reap the benefits. Luckily, science has just shown the exact opposite to be true. According to a 2019 study,[33] when people start to exercise in midlife, even if they have not worked out before, they can rapidly gain most of the benefits of working out, including to the immune system and the brain. However, people who had been active as young adults but sedentary in middle age seemed to lose any associated benefits. That's why I tell my patients that it's never too late to start exercising and make it a daily habit.

THE TYPE OF EXERCISE YOUR CHOOSE MATTERS

The goal of recreational exercise should focus on improving the flow and control of movement. Researchers have known that mastering certain activities demands considerable thought, and consequently, can alter the workings of the brain. Non-contact sports that stress hand-eye coordination and have a low risk of injury, like tennis, golf, or juggling, all require concentration, strategy, and mental attention that enhances overall brain health. Running or jogging and other aerobic activities, while not generally considered cerebral, activate parts of the brain affecting intellectual function and thinking powers, even after the activity is over because they increase CBF.

Yoga, or other stretching exercises, can relieve stress and put you into a meditative state, which has proven brain health benefits, as discussed in chapter 7. Stretching exercises are particularly beneficial to older adults who pose the risk of *sarcopenia*, a term given to age-related muscle loss. Muscle mass decreases approximately 2 percent every year after the age of 50.

If you want to continue to exercise as you get older, resistance training is an effective exercise intervention that prevents sarcopenia later in life. Such training improves gait speed, balance, and stability. Adults should perform resistance training at least 2 to 3 days per week.

Core muscle strength training has been widely studied in relation to the health of the nervous system.[34] The body's core, which represents the connection between the arms and legs, is a separate functional unit in which different muscles interact, including the shoulders and pelvic muscles that are not located in the thoracic-lumbar region.[35] Developing core stability is synonymous with motor control, while enhancing core strength is identified with muscle force.

Those who wish to develop core strength should find a sports trainer to assure a safe experience and to avoid injury. If you want to focus on body and mind synergy, and concentrate on core stability, an excellent choice is the study of Tai Chi. This is an ancient mind-body exercise that utilizes continuous aerobic exercise and strong concentration with breathing control when performed. This combination results in physical benefits such as improvements in aerobic capacity, muscle strength, balance, and motor control, as well as psychological benefits of improved attentiveness, reduced stress and anxiety, and brain health.[36] In one large study of 2,553 individuals age 60 years and older, Tai Chi enhanced cognitive function particularly in executive functioning in individuals without underlying cognitive impairment. Furthermore, a growing body of evidence using magnetic resonance imaging studies suggests that Tai Chi enhances neuroplasticity,[37] and is recommended for those suffering from traumatic brain injury and depression.

9

Survey Your Environment for Toxic Exposures

The fifth and last step in the action plan is to survey your environment, particularly for mold and inadvertent heavy metal exposures. These toxins affect brain health in many different ways and may be contributing to your symptoms. They are so potent that they can even affect epigenetic mechanisms when they are transmitted to babies through breast milk, leading to neurodegenerative diseases that could so easily be averted.

MERCURY

Heavy metals are a category of naturally occurring metals with relatively high densities. Some heavy metals are either essential nutrients (typically iron, cobalt, and zinc) or relatively harmless (such as ruthenium, silver, and indium). Other heavy metals, such as cadmium, mercury, and lead, are highly poisonous. Potential sources of heavy metal poisoning stem from mining, industrial waste, agricultural runoff, paints, and treated timber.

One of the most common heavy metal toxins is mercury. It can be found in old dental fillings and old paint, and it collects in the muscles of sea- and freshwater fish. The mercury that naturally occurs in our atmosphere settles in water, where it is ingested by smaller fish which are eventually consumed by larger fish. Fish at the top of the food chain (e.g., tuna, swordfish, or shark) may have considerable amounts of mercury.

Mercury can pass through the BBB and activate an immune system response, including the production by microglial cells and tumor necrosis factor-α and glutamic acid, both of which are potentially toxic to the brain. Low-grade chronic exposure to mercury induces subtle symptoms including fatigue, anxiety, depression, and short-term memory loss. Subtler clinical findings among dentists who have had chronic mercury exposure include delayed reaction time, poor fine motor control, and deficits in mental concentration. Evidence also links elemental mercury to depression, excessive anger, and anxiety.[1]

At higher exposures, symptoms include changes in coordination, tremors, loss of mental concentration capacity, altered emotional state, and immune dysfunction. Mercury exposure leads to demyelinating peripheral neuropathy on electromyography and nerve conduction studies.[2]

Although there is limited literature regarding mercury toxicity and neurological infectious illness, low doses of elemental mercury have been employed experimentally in two disorders where it alters cell and humor-mediated immune responses: tropical sore (also known as chiclero ulcer, or more formally cutaneous Leishmaniasis) and Lyme disease. These experiments raise the intriguing possibility that symptoms of chronic Lyme disease may be due in part to additional mercury exposure.

LEAD

Lead is another poisonous heavy metal that has been directly linked to neurological dysfunction in adults and children, and can lead to impaired neurobehavioral development. There are clear associations between elevated blood lead levels in children and lower intelligence quotient (IQ) scores,[3] neuropsychological test scores,[4] lower cognitive function, and overall declines in achievement in school.[5] Lead can also directly affect temperament.[6] There is widespread recognition that even low-level exposure alters behavior in young children, including disturbances in memory and learning, visual attention, abstract problem-solving, task switching, and motor dexterity.[7] Of the neurocognitive disruptions identified in low-level lead-exposed children, changes in memory may have the most profound implications for life-long brain health. The brain regions critical for memory and learning, in particular the hippocampus/dentate gyrus regions, overlap neurogenesis pathways. Early disruption of these regions and pathways has the potential to alter neural pathway formation,[8] memory function, learning during development,[9] and neurogenesis,[10] as well as increasing vulnerability to cognitive decline and dementia.

Dust, water, and paint chips are the major sources of lead exposure. Lead is often found in cosmetics, food supplements, food preparation utensils, and improperly prepared infant formula. Diagnosis of lead toxicity has traditionally been based on significantly elevated blood lead levels. However, new research implicates low-level exposures that were previously considered normal as causative factors in cognitive dysfunction, neurobehavioral disorders, and neurological damage.

MOLD

Mold is a type of fungus that grows from tiny spores that float in the air. It can grow almost anywhere the spores land and find moisture and a comfortable temperature, between 40 and 100 degrees Fahrenheit (F). That can include about every damp place in your home.

Toxicity due to mold is a prominent cause of many subtle yet insidious neurological symptoms. Mold mycotoxins, the tiniest parts that are poisonous, originate from the mold fungus. They are so small that there is great difficulty in detecting them in both food and in the atmosphere. They can interfere with cellular mechanisms and can cause inflammation. The route of mold exposure occurs through one of several ways: ingestion, inhalation, or direct contact with mycotoxins. Some people have mold growth inside their bodies that triggers a constant reaction.

The symptoms and signs of chronic mold exposure are wide ranging. In terms of brain health, mold exposure can cause fatigue, neurocognitive symptoms, headache, insomnia, dizziness, anxiety, depression, irritability, tremors, balance disturbance, and autonomic nervous system dysfunction.[11]

Illness resulting from mold exposure can be due to infection, toxicity, allergy, and inflammatory responses triggered by exposure to one or more of the agents present in water-damaged buildings and are often mediated by oxidative stress. Types of disorders that can be seen resulting from water-damaged environments, mold, mycotoxins, and bacteria include involvement of the nervous system through the model of I-Cubed, which asserts that mold infection leads to altered immunity and inflammation. This can lead to infections, sinusitis, allergies, asthma, immune suppression and modulation, autoimmune disorders, mitochondrial toxicity, neurotoxicity, and DNA alterations. Inflammation triggered by exposure also appears to play a significant role in illness during and after exposure to water-damaged environments.[12]

The most common mycotoxins responsible for brain health symptoms are aflatoxins, ochratoxins, and trichothecenes. Aflatoxins can be found in inadequately dry storage units used for peanuts, corn, cotton seed, and grains, and can be transferred onto these foods. Ochratoxins are toxic to the liver and kidney, and have immune suppressant and carcinogenic effects. Like the aflatoxins, they accumulate in fat tissue and are not readily excreted from the body. Common sources of ochratoxins are drying or decaying vegetation, seeds, nuts, and fruits.

Acute toxic exposure to trichothecenes can cause nausea, vomiting, anorexia, headache, abdominal pain, chills, giddiness, and convulsions, whereas chronic exposure can lead to increased susceptibility to microbial infection.

Numerous investigations have demonstrated that fungal materials found inside buildings with moisture damage can lead to systemic inflammation and a risk for acquired illness. Among home inspections of exposed children with evidence of subclinical inflammation, there were increased levels of pro-inflammatory cytokines detected in the blood, particularly when major moisture damage was found in the children's main living areas such as the living room, kitchen, bedroom, and bathroom.[13] In 1989, the Massachusetts Department of Public Health estimated that indoor air pollution accounted for up to 50 percent of all illness[14]; it is likely this has increased since then and it would be expected that water-damaged indoor environments would be a significant contributor.

Meet Lara

Lara is a mid-30s dermatologist who was healthy her entire life until eight years ago, when she first discovered that she could not workout at the gym as usual, as if her muscles just did not have the same strength or endurance. She also developed headaches, imbalance, and difficulty breathing in colder weather or exercising. She also began to have sinus problems, including a chronic stuffy nose with dripping, as well as abdominal discomfort and bloating.

At first Lara wasn't too concerned; after all, she was a doctor. But over the next eight years she met with more than a dozen physicians to try to find the source of these strange new and seemingly progressing symptoms. She went to an integrative doctor who diagnosed her with hypothyroidism and started her on thyroid medication, supplements, and probiotics. She went to ear, nose, and throat, and allergist immunology doctors who found irritation, congestion, and obstructive airway disease. She later developed red swollen skin sensitivities from all the skin testing she had to endure.

When I first met Lara, I noticed that she had vertigo and lightheadedness, and numbness and tingling in the hands and feet. Several months later, body PET imaging showed enlargement of lymph tissue in the lungs, and an endoscopic biopsy showed sarcoidosis, a disease involving abnormal collections of chronic inflammatory cells that form lumps known as granulomas. She also had evidence of orthostatic hypotension on tilt table testing. The cause of sarcoidosis is unknown, but it is believed to result from an abnormally overzealous immune reaction to a trigger such as an infection or chemicals in those who are genetically predisposed.[15] It was unclear how or why this lung disease developed but she was given oral anti-inflammatory medication to quiet down the immune cells that were creating these granulomas in her lungs, but this did not help her symptoms.

Over the next year, she experienced continued deterioration in her health, until it was found that she was suffering from festering mold toxicity. Unknowingly, she had exposed herself to black mold in her apartment that was the likeliest cause of her systemic and neurological illness. At first Lara couldn't believe it, because she lived in a nearly brand-new building. However, she found that there was ongoing water damage, causing mold. She begged her landlord for an entire year to remediate the damage, but to no avail, and she eventually moved to a cleaner and safer building.

I treated Lara with SCIg therapy, which she reports has helped tremendously with all of her neurological symptoms.

DEVELOP A DETOXIFICATION PLAN

Physicians are increasingly being asked to diagnose and treat people suffering from toxic exposures, and I have found a number of approaches that have been proven to help reverse illness caused by these exposures, and ultimately restore health. First, as you've learned, any good treatment must begin by a definitive diagnosis. If you believe that you are suffering from one of these three main sources of environmental toxins, ask your doctor to request the environmental toxin panel of blood and urine levels, and related tissue specimens of hair and nails to search for heavy metal deposits mentioned in chapter 5.

Avoidance alone does not stop mycotoxin-induced disease processes.[16] Affected patients often require other therapies such as intradermal provocative neutralization testing and treatment not only for molds that they actually exposed to, but also to those common in the air. Those with impaired immune systems require an immunomodulatory such as intravenous or subcutaneous immunoglobulin therapy.[17]

Avoid Toxic Foods

Once you've been properly diagnosed, the next course of action is avoidance. Complete removal of mercury- or mold-contaminated foods in your home, and then adopting the practice of not eating them going forward, is the least invasive way to address the issue. I've found that symptoms of mercury toxicity generally subside slowly once people stop eating fish high in mercury; recovery from mold toxicity can take even longer.

According to the Environmental Working Group,[18] the following fish have the highest levels of mercury and should be avoided if you are pregnant, experiencing symptoms, and/or test positively for mercury exposure:

- Bluefin and bigeye tuna steaks or sushi
- Canned light and albacore tuna
- Halibut
- King mackerel
- Lobster
- Mahi mahi
- Marlin
- Orange roughy
- Sea bass
- Shark
- Swordfish
- Tilefish

Remove Mold and Lead in Your Home

Aside from changing your diet, you can limit your toxic exposure drastically by having your home and/or office carefully checked for both mold and lead. You may need to have your home remediated and the offending toxin completely removed. Look for water damage on walls, floors, and furniture for signs of mold. Almost every home gets mold infestations; the trick to mold remediation is to get to them before they get too big. Removing mold can be done with ordinary household cleaning products. But disturbing big infestations on bathroom walls and other places can be bad for your health. When you discover an extensive mold problem, use protective measures (wear special respirators, in addition to goggles and gloves that can be purchased at a hardware store; increase ventilation by using a window fan that you are willing to throw away when you are done, because the spores are almost impossible to clean off; tape plywood or cardboard around window openings so the spores can't blow back in) or hire a professional (you can search "Environmental and Ecological Consultants" online, or call your local public health department).

You can easily spot the most visible type of mold, called mildew, which begins as tiny black spots that can grow into larger colonies. It's the black stuff you see in the grout lines in your shower, on damp walls, and outdoors on the surfaces of deck boards and painted siding, especially in shady areas. If you have a high concentration of mold, you may smell it. If you detect the typical musty odor, check for mold on damp carpets, damp walls, damp crawlspaces and wet wood under your floors, wet roof sheathing, and other damp areas.

A mildewed surface is often difficult to distinguish from a dirty one: to test for mildew, simply dab a few drops of household bleach on the blackened area, and if it lightens after one to two minutes, you have mildew. If the area remains dark, you probably have dirt. Mildew won't damage your home's structure, but other types of mold can cause rot. Remove mildew from wood when you probe the suspect area with a screwdriver or other sharp tool. If the wood is soft or crumbles, the fungi have taken hold and rot has begun.

The key to stopping mold is to control dampness. The worst infestations usually occur in damp crawlspaces, in attics and walls where water has leaked in from the outside, and in basements with poor foundation drainage. You can scrub away surface mold with a 1-to-8 bleach/water cleaning solution. But often mold grows and spreads in places you don't notice, until you spot surface staining, feel mushy drywall, or detect that musty smell. You can also buy mildew cleaner at hardware stores, paint stores, and most home centers. If the mold doesn't disappear after light scrubbing, reapply the cleaning mix and let it sit for another minute or two. Then lightly scrub again. Lastly, seal the clean surfaces when they're thoroughly dry to slow future moisture penetration. Apply a grout sealer (available at tile shops and home centers) to tile joints to thwart mold regrowth.

Your home or office may have lead paint if it was built before 1978, even if it has been repainted. Follow the same protective procedures for mold removal. Work on one room at a time. This technique is a complete removal of all lead paint from the underlying surface. Mist surfaces with water while using hand scrapers to dislodge the paint.

Chelation

Once the contaminated areas in your home have been addressed, you may find that you are still feeling the effects of toxins. The next step in treatment involves a comprehensive approach utilizing nutritional and detoxification strategies.

Chelation is the conventional recommendation for removing lead and mercury. This therapy pulls heavy metals out of the body's tissue and into the bloodstream, where it can be removed. Chelation is always administered by a healthcare provider.

Sequestering agents find toxins in the gastrointestinal tract, thus reducing recirculation. These agents are not absorbed into systemic circulation; therefore, side effects are typically limited to gastrointestinal symptoms and potential malabsorption of medications and nutrients, especially if the dose is poorly timed. Sequestering agents have a large surface-area-to-volume ratio, giving large absorptive capacity. Several agents that have shown specific efficacy in lowering mycotoxin and endotoxin levels, including cholestyramine, activated carbons, and chlorella, are prescribed by your doctor and taken at home under physician supervision. Additionally, these agents are non-specific and can bind additional toxins, helping to lower total body burden of toxins. Of course, they have the potential to bind medications, vitamins, and nutrients and should be taken several hours apart from medications and vitamins and ideally on an empty stomach.

Nutritional Supplements and Foods that Heal

If you believe that you've been exposed to lead, studies suggest that taking specific vitamins and generally upping your intake of vegetables and fruit may help support detoxification.[19] Vitamin C, B1, and B6 deficiencies have been reported to enhance sensitivity toward lead toxicity.[20] Common deficiencies encountered include vitamin D, magnesium, zinc, and coenzyme Q10, all of which can adversely affect multiple pathways in the body necessary for detoxi-fication, thereby perpetuating the effects of the toxin exposure.

What's more, vitamin supplementation has proved to be effective against lead toxicity in both human and animal studies. Vitamins C and E are antioxi-dants that are able to scavenge free radicals. Vitamin B1 has been reported to decrease lead levels in the liver, kidneys, bone, and blood by increasing excre-tion.[21] Vitamin B6 has also been found to be effective in reducing accumula-tion of lead in tissues, a function that has been attributed to the ring nitrogen atom in its structure, which can naturally chelate lead before it is absorbed into the body.[22] These dietary supplements are affordable, with fewer side ef-fects than chelation therapy.[23]

Vegetables, fruits, and other edible plants are important dietary sources of vitamins and essential minerals that can decrease the risks of lead toxicity. Plants in particular provide a wide variety of nutrients, such as dietary pro-tein and phytochemicals, which have been reported to have beneficial effects against lead toxicity. For example, green tea and curry spices are commonly used in Asian cooking and are thought to alleviate oxidative stress.[24]

The following can act as natural antagonists to lead toxicity and should be consumed daily if you believe you are suffering from environmental toxins:

- Berries
- Curry spices
- Garlic
- Grapes
- Green tea
- Onions
- Tomatoes

Investigate Probiotics

Probiotics are bacterial supplements that contain live microorganisms which, when administered in adequate amounts, may have considerable health benefits. The most common are *Lactobacillus* and *Bifidobacterium*. Over the years, the scientific interest to discover, assess, and analyze species with probiotic properties has intensively grown. There are a significant number of studies indicating the benefits of probiotics in relation to antibiotic-associated diarrhea, allergy, lactose intolerance, reduction of cholesterol, as well as devel-opment of immune system and protection against gut pathogens.[25] Probiotics have been studied for their modulating effects of toxins, including mold myco-toxins. These treatments have the potential to have significant beneficial effects as much of the metabolism of toxins occurs via intestinal biotransformation.

Some species are known to have antioxidative properties,[26] which may be another important characteristic for heavy metal toxicity protection.

Sweating Out Toxins

Sauna and other forms of sweat induction have been used safely in many cultures throughout history and have long been studied as a means of reducing our toxic load.[27] The most frequently studied saunas are Finnish dry heat radiant saunas, although infrared saunas are also used effectively and have the advantage of inducing sweating at a lower body temperature.

BOX 9.1

LOWERING INFLAMMATION
IS A LIFELONG PROCESS

The TAPES protocol may help you reverse many of your brain health symptoms. However, lowering inflammation is a beneficial practice that you can follow for the rest of your life. This doesn't mean that you will need to take medications forever, but you can continue to follow the detoxification and eating recommendations long after you are feeling better. In fact, the best advice is to follow the protocol as a combination of preventative measures and treating infections as they occur.

THE NEXT STEP

Now that you understand all of the components of the TAPES protocol, you can begin to put these in action. Based on your testing/quiz results from chapter 5, you can skip to the chapter in part III that is most closely aligned with your symptoms. There, you'll find information that explains what you are experiencing and specific tips to help you reverse your condition.

III

AUTOIMMUNE DISEASES THAT AFFECT BRAIN HEALTH

Developmental Disorders Affecting Children and Teens

One of the most harrowing experiences for any parent is to have a child that appears healthy, yet is not thriving or has noticeable neurobehavioral or neuropsychiatric symptoms. No matter the child's age, parents can be frustrated, scared, and confused by their children's poor health. Sometimes, changes to the behavior or thinking seem to come out of nowhere and look like obsessive-compulsive behaviors, suicidal thoughts, tics, and/or mood swings reminiscent of bipolar disorder. Other times, symptoms can be progressive.

I see parents of such children regularly, and no matter how old their child is, they are often concerned that their son or daughter's brain health blips will lead to some type of permanent mental deficiency if left unchecked. Their worries include mental retardation, learning disabilities, long-lasting neuropsychiatric tendencies, or mental illness. In many instances, these parents are correct, and ultimately, that's good news. We now know that if problems with neural development are caught early, the trajectory toward illness may be altered by treatment for the specific disease aided by innate neural plasticity that remodels brain circuits.

I tell these patients all the time that they need to be the best advocates for their children. I urge them to read up on the real science of what their child may be experiencing, and not just to enter keywords into search engines and read the horror stories often found on the internet. Then, once they are well-versed, they are in a much better position to explore different medical options. This is the time to join an internet or social media group of parents facing similar concerns. These groups have proven to be incredibly useful. First, the parent will quickly be able to find out that their child's illness is not all that uncommon. They'll hear about new treatments and learn firsthand how they were tolerated.

Most importantly, don't wait for your child to come to you. Many times, children and teens will not have the language to express how they are feeling or the changes they're experiencing. Often, they simply do not have the capacity to ask their parents, "Am I okay?" even when they can tell something is wrong. Children and teens who feel unwell will become *involutional*, which means they start looking inwards for the answer, subsequently blaming themselves as the cause of the problem. As parents, we need to pay attention, look for the warning signals, and then act on their behalf.

If your child is suffering from brain health symptoms, this chapter may provide the answers you've been searching for. Please share this information with your child's doctors. If you find that they aren't open to new ideas, it may be time to reevaluate the relationship and find someone more willing to explore new trends and treatments. Whatever you do, don't throw in the towel with your child's health. If after a year, you haven't made gains with their psychiatric status, you may very well be dealing with a neuropsychiatric problem which may be related to I-Cubed.

The following sections review, in age order, some of the most common developmental disorders that I see that can be linked to infection, inflammation, and immunity.

AUTISM: A DEVELOPMENTAL DISORDER INFLUENCED BY AUTOIMMUNITY

Most adults with autism know that they have a disorder, so new brain health symptoms are not likely to be caused by an onset of adult autism. However, I've had many frantic mothers come to see me when their very young children have a sudden or progressive change in behavior.

Autism is a pervasive developmental disorder and is usually apparent by the age of 3. Autism spectrum disorder (ASD) is the name for the broader range of autistic behaviors. ASD shows a striking sex bias with a male:female ratio ranging from 4:1 to 10:1.

The entire spectrum of autism is characterized by a triad of brain health symptoms:[1]

- Limited or absent verbal communication
- Lack of reciprocal social interaction or responsiveness
- Restricted stereotypic and ritualized patterns of interests and behavior

Many researchers currently believe that the underlying cause of autism includes the contribution of inflammatory-autoimmune insults that trigger abnormal neuronal development. Recent research out of Columbia University shows that there is a real correlation between intestinal microbes and autism. This line of thinking originated with Andrew Wakefield, who was doing research in intestinal microbiology in the late 1990s,[2,3] when he found that children with autism also had intestinal viral products embedded in their intestinal walls, especially in the lymph glands.

There is no shortage of hypotheses to explain the observed association between ASD and gastrointestinal (GI) disturbances. One commonly held explanation is that GI dysfunction is a secondary effect or byproduct of ASD behavior, specifically food selectivity. Although it has been shown that the diets of children with ASD quickly diverge from the norm, overall nutritional intake has not been shown to differ and a nutritional profile associated with GI habits in ASD has not yet been found.[4] Other explanations include shared genetic factors[5] and shared mechanisms of the development of both disorders, including those that involve innate immunity,[6] the role of microbes and autoimmunity in neuropsychiatric illness,[7] impaired metabolism,[8] and compromised neurotransmitter signaling in the brains of affected children.[9] One study examining patients with ASD indicated that lower GI symptoms, including abdominal pain, stool retention, and large bowel movements, correlated with an elevated level of serotonin in the blood, which was almost entirely derived from the gut in a full one-third of patients.[10,11]

The possibility that the GI tract is not just an innocent bystander in ASD, but a part of its underlying cause, is associated with the "leaky gut" hypothesis. Affected individuals with defects in intestinal epithelial barrier permeability manifest inappropriate signaling by the enteric bacteria, environmental toxins, and even dietary macromolecules that then pass through the epithelial barrier and into the bloodstream.[12] This hypothesis is one reason why I recommend that people with CNS disorders follow the diet suggestions in chapter 5, which are meant to heal and seal the gut wall and improve intestinal function.[13]

Although a link between altered immune responses and ASD was first recognized nearly 40 years ago, only recently has new evidence started to shed
light on the complex multifaceted relationship between immune dysfunction
and behavior.[7] There are now several lines of evidence that point to altered
immune dysfunction in ASD. Extensive alterations in immune function have
now been described in both children and adults with ASD, including ongoing
inflammation in the brain, elevated pro-inflammatory cytokine profiles in the
cerebral spinal fluid and blood, increased presence of brain-specific autoantibodies, and altered immune cell function.

Microbes in the gut can induce autoantibodies that bind to the brain and
affect behavior, and specifically the CNS.[8] An increased prevalence of family members who all suffer from some form of autoimmunity is common
in disorders as diverse as schizophrenia, obsessive-compulsive disorder,
and autism, and suggests that differences in exposure timing and genetic
vulnerability toward autoimmunity are important determinants of neuropsychiatric outcomes.

Autistic children show evidence of alterations of their own intestinal barrier and increased T-cell activation in the intestinal mucosa. These changes
may contribute to the development of autism. Even though GI symptoms
are common in early childhood, children with ASD may experience more
GI difficulties in the first 3 years of life than children with normal or delayed
development. Treatments that address GI symptoms may significantly contribute to the well-being of children with ASD and may be useful in reducing difficult behaviors. What's more, intestinal complaints of ASD children
seem to run in the family. New research based on the Norwegian Mother
and Child Cohort Study[14] (a longitudinal study tracking 90,000 pregnant
women from 1998 to 2008) showed that maternally reported GI symptoms
were more common for mothers of ASD children than in mothers with children of typical development.

The Autism Birth Cohort[15] was established to explore genetic and pre- or
perinatal environmental factors, as well as the interplay between genes and
environment, and to facilitate discovery of biomarkers with potential to enable early recognition and treatment. Apart from the impact of infection and
autoimmunity, ASD has been associated with increased maternal (over 35
years at the time of pregnancy)[16] or paternal age (over 40 year at the time of
pregnancy),[17] use of medications during pregnancy, children with low birth

weight and congenital malformations,[18] underlying genetic factors and obstetric complications,[19] and maternal exposure to drugs and substance abuse.[20] These potential risk factors may each trigger the aberrant neuronal development characterizing autism.

AUTISM'S INCREASED PREVALENCE AND THE VACCINATION CONTROVERSY

The prevalence of childhood autism and ASD has increased 20- to 30-fold in epidemiological studies in the decades leading up to 2000, estimating a prevalence rise from 1 in 2500 children (0.04 percent)[21,22] in the late 1960s to 2 percent of vaccination-eligible age children.[23]

Back in the 1990s, there was a lay group of British moms who believed that certain vaccinations caused autism. Researcher Andrew Wakefield[24,25] believed that the viral products were derived from vaccinations, yet his theory has since been disproven and thoroughly discounted. A separate case-control study[26] found that vaccinated children with autism and GI disturbances were no more likely than age-matched children undergoing clinically indicated ileo-colonoscopy to have measles virus RNA or inflammation in bowel tissues, nor was the onset of autism or GI disturbances temporally related to receipt of a MMR vaccine. Interestingly, measles vaccine virus (MeVV) RNA were found in ileal biopsy tissue of one boy with autism and GI disturbances and reactive small and large intestine lymphoid follicles.

TREATING AUTISM

There is no cure for ASD, and there's no medication currently available to treat it. There are medicines that can help with related brain health symptoms, including depression, seizures, insomnia, and difficulty focusing. Behavioral therapies, in combination with medicines, have shown promise. Some of the most cutting-edge ASD research currently focuses on the potential benefit of IVIg therapy.[27,28]

Some ASD children respond positively to the TAPES protocol, including dietary intervention, avoiding allergic foods, and managing environmental factors, such as identifying and removing mold from the home. For example, one of the mothers in my practice often says, "My child was definitely diagnosed as autistic, and then I adjusted his diet and gave him antibiotics, and he became normal again."

Autistic children often display disruptive behavior and noncompliance. Several evidence-based behavioral interventions are available, such as parent-child interaction therapy (PCIT). The overarching focus of this therapy is to positively reframe the caregiver-child relationship using conditioning techniques and play therapy.[29] The results of recent research[30] shows that PCIT significantly improves parent-reported disruptive behavior in children with ASD at levels comparable to children without ASD. In another study of children and caregivers,[31] significant improvements were found in parents' self-reported emotion dysregulation, and their self-report of children's symptoms, parenting practices, and reflective functioning in the form of "prementalizing," meaning their capacity to understand the emotional world of their child. What's more, PCIT seems to address the sleep problems commonly associated with autistic children.[32]

Meet Will

Will was a 5-year-old boy when I first met him. His parents brought him to see me because he was not thriving. Since the age of 2 he slept poorly, often for only a few hours a night, and had severe separation anxiety. By the time he came to see me, Will had developed many of the autistic warning signs: he had lost much of his language skills and was becoming increasingly asocial.

Will also had a history of recurrent autoimmune conditions, including bacterial infections, sinus infections, gastroesophageal reflux, hypothyroidism, and Crohn disease. He had been diagnosed with common variable immune deficiency syndrome, a disorder that impairs the immune system. People with common variable immune deficiency (CVID) syndrome are highly susceptible to infection from bacteria, viruses, and often develop recurrent infections, particularly in the lungs, sinuses, and ears. In addition, he did not react to a polysaccharide challenge that tested his ability to clear effectively with encapsulated bacterial organisms responsible for chronic upper respiratory infection.

I started Will on an antibiotic regimen followed by IVIg. We also ran food allergy testing and removed reactive foods from his diet. Over the next 2 years, we carefully monitored him, and while there were a few occasions of heightened agitation and fearful and combative behavior, there were marked improvement in his language and social interactions, followed by gains in learning and memory retention. Today, Will is finished with his IVIg therapy and continues to show increases in his cognition. Happily, his parents report that he is even able to take a bus to school on his own.

There are many autistic children like Will who also have pediatric autoimmune neuropsychiatric disorder associated with group A beta hemolytic streptococcus infections (PANDAS). My research has shown that these children often manifest fluctuating behavioral symptoms and decreased cognitive skills following infectious and immune insults.[33] Many have similar responses to polysaccharide challenges,[34] and these children are likely candidates for IVIg supplementation. Sometimes, these children are erroneously diagnosed with specific antibody deficiency or partial antibody deficiency and impaired polysaccharide responsiveness.

ADOLESCENT BEHAVIORAL CHANGES

The term "adolescence" is generally used to describe a transition stage between childhood and adulthood. For our purposes, adolescence will include both the teenage years and puberty, as these terms are not mutually exclusive.

The brain is constantly changing during the adolescent years, which is why is it considered to be one of the most dynamic events of human growth and development, second only to infancy. These changes are similar to that noticed during infancy and consist of a thickening of the gray matter as well as an increase in the total number of neurons, or brain cells. This neuronal rewiring continues from the onset of puberty up until 24 years old, and most notably affects the prefrontal cortex, which is the decision-making region of the brain. The rewiring is accomplished through two different tasks: dendritic pruning and myelination. Dendritic pruning eliminates unused synapses and is generally considered a beneficial process, and myelination increases the speed of impulse conduction across the brain's region-specific neural circuitry. The myelination also optimizes the communication of information throughout the CNS and augments the speed of information processing. These changes strengthen a young adult's ability to multitask, solve problems, and process complex information. This changing brain provides the necessary abilities to develop talents and life-long interests.

Out of several neurotransmitters produced in the CNS, two play a significant role in the maturation of adolescent behavior: dopamine and serotonin. Dopamine influences brain events that control movement, emotional response, and the ability to experience pleasure and pain. Its levels decrease during adolescence, resulting in mood swings and difficulties regulating emotions. Serotonin plays a significant role in mood alterations, anxiety, impulse control, and arousal. Its levels also decrease during adolescence, and this is associated with decreased impulse control. New evidence suggests that another neurotransmitter, gamma-aminobutyric acid (GABA), which affects the prefrontal cortex, remains under construction during adolescence. This may be responsible for neurobehavioral excitement including euphoria and risk-taking behavior like reckless driving, unprotected sex, and drug abuse. In fact, most drug addictions initiate during adolescence.

Brain maturation is also governed by several other factors, including heredity and environment, history of prenatal and postnatal insult, nutritional status, sleep patterns, and medications the adolescent may be taking. Other variables include physical, mental, economical, and psychological stress; illicit substance use, and alcohol intake. Changes in sex hormone production, including estrogen, progesterone, and testosterone, all influence the development and maturation of the adolescent brain.

When teens experience brain health issues, one of the first clues may be neurobehavioral. The most obvious can be *tics*, which are rapid, repetitive movements or vocal utterances and obsessive-compulsive disorder (OCD) behaviors. Tics can involve the body, like excessive eye blinking, the voice, such as a habitual cough or throat clearing, and can both come and go, or become chronic. Tics are often mistaken for the fidgety signs of attention deficit hyperactivity disorder, yet they are different, in that they usually involve rapid, repeated, identical movements. When otherwise normal children develop these symptoms, I search for a variety of causes that falls under the rubrics of infectious, metabolic, autoimmune, genetic, dietary, or structural brain changes. Watching and waiting while investigating the possibilities seems like a wise approach. For example, my friend Greg's son was going through a period in high school where he was lining up his pencils, grinding his teeth, had pain in his jaw, and at the same time had to go on antibiotics for some sinus infection. The OCD behaviors went away. Genuine and functional tics are observed in teen girls who follow TikTok and other social media platforms that personify them.

Another common manifestation of brain dysfunction of particular importance are obsessive-compulsive or obsessive-compulsive–like behaviors. According to the Mayo Clinic, OCD refers to a pattern of unreasonable thoughts and fears (obsessions) that can lead to repetitive behaviors (compulsions) and elaborate rituals. These obsessions and compulsions can range from mild (lining up pencils on a desk) to severe (excessing handwashing). As these symptoms become more complex, they can interfere with daily activities and cause significant distress. Disturbances of neuronal circuits may be the basis of obsessive-compulsive behaviors routinely seen in adolescents, either in response to maturational challenges in the nervous system, dysfunction of brain circuitry, or abnormalities in brain activation and connectivity.[35]

Glutamate, dopamine, and serotonin neurotransmission have all been implicated in OCD.[36] There are beneficial effects of SSRIs for treating OCD, even though the exact mechanism of action remains elusive.[37] An autoimmune hypothesis for the development of an OCD subtype has also been suggested, implicating group A beta-hemolytic streptococcal (GABHS) infection in PANDAS. This subgroup manifests changes in antistreptococcal, antineuronal, or antibasal ganglia antibody titers, immune cells, and circulating cytokines.[38] I have also observed many instances in which young children, and especially young adults in high school and college, may be affected by an autoimmune disorder that is causing their brain health symptoms. For instance, I recently treated a 16-year-old girl with severe dysautonomia, a malfunction of the autonomic nervous system, and Lyme disease. One of the first things her mother told me was that she had OCD behaviors beginning a year before. My job was to then figure out the timeline of her illness so that we could prescribe the right treatment.

The symptoms of OCD include both obsessive and compulsive behaviors, including:

- Arranging items to face a certain way
- Constant checking
- Constant counting
- Fear of contamination
- Impulsive behaviors
- Persistent sexual thoughts
- Repeated unwanted ideas
- Repeatedly cleaning one or more items
- Repeatedly washing hands
- Thoughts that you might be harmed
- Thoughts that you might cause others harm

TREATING OBSESSIVE-COMPULSIVE BEHAVIORS AND TICS

Tics are sudden, non-rhythmic motor movements or vocalizations that are relatively common among school-age children for brief periods of time.[39] However, when tics become an ongoing issue or interfere with school or family life, parents should investigate. The symptoms of tics that typically emerge in early childhood may remit in some children, even those with chronic tic disorders, such as Tourette disorder. Adolescents who develop tics may find that they persist into adulthood.[40] Untreated, common tics that include eye blinking, head jerking, mouth movements, and simple vocalizations can lead to considerable impairment for those affected, and they could diminish quality of life.[41]

Historically, tics have been managed with antipsychotic medications known as neuroleptics such as fluoxetine (Prozac) and autonomic adrenergic receptor stimulants such as clonidine (Catapres).[42] Although effective, these medications are often accompanied by significant side effects, so much so that I find that my patients and their parents often express a preference for non-pharmacological treatments. Behavioral interventions such as habit reversal training and comprehensive behavioral intervention for tics[43] offer excellent alternatives. Both of these therapies include awareness training and competing response training.[44]

Meet Darnelle

Most kids that develop a neurologic illness frequently develop OCD as well. For example, in the 18 months preceding Darnelle's visit to me, this 8-year-old girl had manifested tics, OCD, and attention deficit hyperactivity disorder (ADHD) behaviors, included screaming, curling of her fingers and toes, and focus issues. Another doctor had suggested that her behaviors may be linked to an earlier prescription of Lexapro, which had been used to treat her anxiety. She was seen by a pediatric allergist immunologist who found markedly elevated levels of circulating cytokines consistent with autoimmunity. Darnelle had also been given antibiotics to treat what was thought to be a Lyme infection, because she had vacationed in a Lyme endemic area, yet a course of prednisone seemed to provide more benefit.

When I examined Darnelle, I found that she had incredible autonomic changes and some peripheral neuropathy. Magnetic resonance imaging fused with positron emission tomography showed linear signal changes in the subcortical left peri-atrial white matter, most likely in areas of terminal myelination, with frontal lobe white matter changes and areas of hypo-metabolism in the hippocampi. There was similar diffuse hypometabolism throughout the brain stem and cerebellum. I also diagnosed tics and OCD as a manifestation of autoimmune encephalopathy.

We began treatment right away, including a year of weekly IVIg therapy, cognitive behavioral therapy, and clonidine (Catapres) to address her tics. The current first-line treatment for OCD includes cognitive behavioral therapy (CBT); however, I find that about 60 percent of patients respond to this treatment, and even among responders symptoms often persist.

A year later, our follow-up positron emission tomography magnetic resonance imaging showed complete resolution of the brain changes. Darnelle's tics decreased, and so did her OCD behaviors.

11

Sore Throats Lead to Sore Heads

On the Lookout for PANDAS and PANS

PANDAS and PANS are post-infectious autoimmune (I-Cubed) neuropsychiatric disorders; however, PANDAS occurs uniquely in association with group A beta-hemolytic streptococcal infections (GABHS). Both are as complex as they sound. These are childhood neuropsychiatric disorders caused by post-infectious autoimmune changes in the brain. As you've learned, your immune system is a complex network of cells, tissues, and organs that work together to defend against foreign invaders to the body, including infections, viruses, and germs. Its job is to keep them out, or if it cannot, the immune system finds and destroys them. However, when the immune system is bombarded with a particular strain of strep throat, tonsillitis, pharyngitis, and ear infections,[1] the infection unleashes an autoimmune response in the brain in some children. I like to think of this mechanism like the way one rude or humiliating comment can pattern your behavior toward that person for months or years later. The immune system operates like that, by holding on to a memory or event, and keeping the struggle alive until the battle is won, and maybe overreacting in the process.

An antibody is then generated through the exposure to strep or to other infections, which then makes its way from the blood circulation into the brain where it attacks the gray matter in what we call the subcortical brain, where movement disorders are seen.

The autoimmune response to GABHS has been the best studied in regards to systemic rheumatic diseases; however, other bacteria and even viruses[2] (as many as 104 different strains), as well as *Mycoplasma pneumonia*[3] and *B. burgdorferi*,[4] the agent of Lyme disease, can all be likely culprits in PANS. These antibodies are thought to be the cause of the brain symptoms. However, there's no way to tell that in fact they are, because there are so many possible infections, and the best test to link any or all of them is to biopsy the brain and see if the tissue reacts to testing. That is what researchers did more than a decade ago in trying to sort out whether all cases of strep throat lead to PANDAS, or just some. The investigators[5] looked at two groups of children, a PANDAS group, comprised with clinically active tics and obsessive-compulsive disorder (OCD), and a GABHS control group of active GABHS infection confirmed by throat culture and elevated antistreptolysin O (ASO) and anti-DNAse B antibody titers but without a history or clinical evidence of tics and OCD. They observed positive antibasal ganglia staining in two-thirds of children with PANDAS and strep throat due to GABHS, but in only 10 percent of the strep throat control group without PANDAS, suggesting that antibrain antibodies present in children with PANDAS could not be explained merely by a history of GABHS infection. If fact, it supported the I-Cubed hypothesis that GABHS turns the immune system on the host through the creation of antibrain antibodies. In that sense, the strep infection is not the direct cause, but a link in the chain of post-infectious autoimmunity.

Children with comprised immune systems, like highly allergic children and those with preexisting sinus infections and recurrent strep throats, are most at risk for developing PANDAS and PANS. However, symptoms of PANDAS and PANS include a sudden onset of tics and OCD-like behavior in an otherwise healthy child. Symptoms can also include pronounced attention deficit disorder, oppositional defiant disorder, depression, sleep anxiety, overanxiousness, bed-wetting, emotional changes, school performance changes, personality changes, bedtime fears, fidgetiness, separation fears, impulsivity, and distraction. It's only when the tics and OCD begin to disturb family dynamics and their progress at school, if they're in school, that teachers and parents notice.

Parents often report that all of a sudden, their child starts lining up their pencils, performing repetitive movements like handwashing, or displaying protective behavior as in yelling, "Stay out of my room. Don't touch my stuff." These behaviors can disturb family dynamics and a child's progress at school, and only seem to get better when the child is treated with a course of antibiotics for a totally unrelated problem, like a sinus infection.

For children who have recurrent sinus infections that are treated with antibiotics, the tics and OCD behavior might wane while they're on antibiotics, but then reoccur when they're off again. However, because the symptoms can be inconsistent, they are often confused with periods of relapses and remissions of a psychological issue, as opposed to a steady decline in physical health. Some doctors will treat the infections in an effort to alter the behavior. For example, if a child had repeated strep infections, the doctor puts them on penicillin suppressive therapies. Some children have their tonsils and adenoids taken out to reduce the number of infections that cause these behaviors. Often, pediatricians will recognize PANDAS for what it is. However, if a pediatrician notices the OCD behavior but does not make the leap to PANDAS, the child may be sent to see a behavioral therapist or put on anti-anxiety medications. They may also be mistaken for Tourette syndrome. Affected children initially misdiagnosed with Tourette syndrome may improve with anti-anxiety and antidepressants, and even cognitive behavioral therapy. However, these children will still experience an overall decline in health because they are not on the proper medications.

Worse, when PANDAS and PANS are misdiagnosed, unfortunately for the child, at some point their OCD behavior becomes accepted as normal. The truth is, dozens of children in every school, every year, are misdiagnosed as behavior problems or having primary psychiatric disease when in fact they have PANDAS or PANS. If the behavior is severe enough to warrant a doctor's visit, and a pediatrician notices the OCD behavior but does not make the leap to diagnose PANDAS, the child may be mismanaged. The most well-intentioned pediatrician might suggest a child psychiatrist who might or might not notice the PANDAS or the PANS, and fail to perform appropriate testing to confirm the real nature of the illness as a process that unfolds in the brain.

TESTING AND TREATING PANDAS AND PANS

Elevated ASO and DNAse B antibody levels provide a marker of this inherent autoimmunity and can distinguish likely cases of PANDAS and PANS. However, false-positive high titers can occur[6] due to sustained high titers result from re-infection, slower rates of the decline in the antibody rise, and a more potent immune response in any given child.[7] The Cunningham panel[8] is an excellent test to begin with, and your doctor can order it if you feel your child is experiencing PANDAS symptoms.[9,10] Normal titers would be useful in excluding PANDAS in a child with new-onset tics and OCD, and negative cultures and/or normal ASO titers, whereas high titers would support PANDAS in a child with culture-positive strep throat and/or elevated ASO and DNAse B levels in the blood.

I have found that immune-modulatory therapy, like IVIg therapy, benefits most affected children.[11] My research builds on earlier discoveries, beginning in 1995, when Allen and colleagues[12] described the first reported successful treatment, employing plasma exchange, immunosuppressive doses of prednisone, and IVIg in conjunction with penicillin. In 2006, Hersh and colleagues[13] reported success with a child with PANDAS in whom immunologic evaluation disclosed low immunoglobulin (Ig)G2/IgG4 subclass levels, suboptimal response to pneumococcal vaccine and rapid decline of pneumococcal antibody titers with low levels of pro-inflammatory cytokines.

When I was a master's student in epidemiology at Columbia University in 2016, I was looking for a thesis project that involved a rich database to analyze. I happened upon Dr. Denis Bouboulis, an allergist and immunologist in Darien, Connecticut, who had noted a favorable impact of IVIg on the neuropsychiatric manifestations of PANDAS and on impaired humoral deficiency in his patients. I took the data from Bouboulis, who treated 150 children with PANDAS who had already received their maximal antibiotic regimen and still had PANDAS symptoms. With his permission and that of the Institutional Review Board of Columbia University's School of Public Health, I de-identified the cases to ensure patient confidentiality, and coded his notes and analyzed them looking at baseline levels of IgG, IgA, and IgM, and subclass levels. My thesis study[14] showed that two-thirds of children with PANDAS improved their symptoms of tics, OCD, and neuropsychiatric behaviors, while 20 percent achieved remission at 12-month follow-up. I also found that children with low baseline levels of total IgG or IgA and their subclasses predicted full remission at 12 months independent of other factors. This study[15] as published in the medical literature stands as the largest series of PANDAS children treated with IVIg to date.[16]

This research presents a strong argument for the efficacy of gamma globulin. We now know that by delivering more and putting more antibodies into the body, IVIg not only resets the immune system—it stabilizes it. It may also be acting by blocking antibodies from attacking the brain. Therefore, IVIg should be part of the multimodal therapeutic approach in children with moderate to severe symptoms of PANDAS and PANS.

In addition to IVIg, patients should receive prophylactic antibiotics to prevent future infection-triggered symptoms. They should also receive standard neuropsychiatric care, including the same medications that lessen OCD and tics (see chapter 10), as well as cognitive-behavior therapy. I also find that mold remediation helps: there are many times where there is unsuspected mold exposure that appears to predate and coincide with the onset of PANDAS and PANS. By treating the underlying mechanism of post-infectious autoimmunity instead of the symptoms alone, we can treat PANS and PANDAS correctly.

BOX 11.1

FOR MORE INFORMATION

The PANDAS Physicians Network (www.pandasppn.org) is an excellent resource. This website presents a systematic graduated approach to treatment of PANDAS and PANS based on the "best practice" standards of expert clinicians from across the United States. In addition to providing suggestions for recognition and diagnosis of PANDAS and PANS, it also offers guidance in the management of patients with varying levels of severity.

Meet Carlos

According to his pediatrician, Carlos had an episode of very bad behavioral changes in 2012 when he struck his mother several times and spit at his father. At the time, he was 7 years old and like most children his age he had developed a severe strep pharyngitis infection. He was treated with azithromycin, and while his throat felt better, his behavior continued to be erratic and violent. His parents consulted a child psychiatrist who treated him with fluoxetine (Prozac) but that was complicated by emotional side effects. A neurologist later placed him on methylphenidate (Concerta), a popular medication used to treat attention deficit disorder (as well as attention deficit hyperactivity disorder), which led to improvement that lasted even after he was taken off the medication. Carlos continued taking Concerta for the next five years, and his behavior seemed to return to normal. Yet on the last day of summer camp in 2017, he came down with strep throat again. Seemingly out of nowhere, Carlos went wild, and by the time he returned home, he was having repeated vocal tics. He was also oppositional and refused to go to back to school, and he was up all night with rage.

Confused and frustrated, Carlos's parents brought him to see me. I ordered an MRI of the brain and spine that was normal. He tested positively for Lyme disease, and we noted through his bloodwork that he was genetically predisposed to Celiac disease. Electrodiagnostic studies showed acquired distal demyelinating changes. Autonomic studies dated showed orthostatic intolerance with hypotension and reflex tachycardia with head-up tilting for 5 minutes. PET/MRI showed glucose hypometabolism in both medial temporal lobes of the brain. I placed him on doxycycline for one month to get rid of his Lyme infection and encouraged Carlos's mother to help him follow a low salt, gluten-free diet. We also started him on IVIg therapy. After 3 months of treatment, Carlos was able to return to school and has since been the sweet boy his parents recognize.

This case demonstrates an important and emerging concept, which is the overlap of cases of PANDAS and PANS with autoimmune encephalitis.[17] Future studies of affected children, meticulously diagnosed and carefully studied, serving as candidates for immune-modulatory therapy incorporating IVIg, plasma exchange, and other immunological approaches, will soon provide measurable direction in the optimal management of PANDAS and PANS.

12

The Gut-Brain Connection

Celiac Disease and Beyond

There is an inextricable relationship that the gut has with the brain. The relationship between the gut and the brain is bidirectional: the gut sends messages to the brain, and the brain sends messages to the gut. The brain–gut connection works on two levels. First, the gut holds the largest number of neurotransmitter receivers outside of the brain. Second, 70 percent of your entire immune system resides in the gut. If you feel depressed or anxious, you may be experiencing a neurotransmitter imbalance that started in your gut. In fact, 90 percent of all the serotonin (a critical hormone associated with mood and social behavior, appetite and digestion, sleep, memory, and sexual desire and function) you make is stored and produced in your gut, not in your brain.

Dr. Tom O'Bryan is a world-renowned expert in gluten sensitivity, and he believes, as I do, that anytime you're dealing with a brain health concern, the first place you can address is the gut. His book, *You Can Fix Your Brain*,[1] talks in detail about the relationship between the gut and the brain. It's recommended reading for anyone who has been diagnosed with gluten sensitivity.

Since we already know how the brain functions, let's look more closely at the gut and how it works. The gut is an organ system that covers every aspect of digestion. Imagine your gut is one long coiled tube—20 to 25 feet—that starts at your mouth and ends at your anus. The food you eat enters the tube and then is broken down into very small pieces (digestion). These pieces have to fit through the lining inside the tube (absorption) in order to get into the bloodstream, where your body uses these particles as the raw materials to make new cells.

The intestines are where the hard work of digestion takes place. They are lined with *microvilli,* microscopic cellular membrane bulges that form the primary surface of nutrient absorption. The intestines are also covered by the *intestinal epithelium,* a single layer of cells that separates the contents of the intestines from the body. The epithelium acts as a barrier, preventing the entry of foreign invaders into the bloodstream. In many ways it is similar to the blood–brain barrier (BBB). It also acts as a selective filter that helps the distribution of nutrients and various other beneficial substances from the intestines to the rest of the body. Yet sometimes the epithelium gets torn, primarily due to inflammation. When this happens, larger molecules can pass through and enter the bloodstream, causing an autoimmune reaction. The immune system addresses these large molecules as if they were foreign invaders and starts the immune response. And when these large molecules travel through the bloodstream up to your brain, they pass through the BBB and affect brain health.

A second issue is the relationship between brain hormones and the microbes—the bacteria, fungi, and viruses—that live in your gut. This community of microbes is called your gut's *microbiome.* The gut's microbiome is almost ten times greater than all the cells in the human body put together. There are also endemic microbiomes of the skin and in each of our organs. A primary function of the gut's microbiome is the development, regulation, and maintenance of the epithelium. It is also linked to manufacturing vitamins, regulating metabolism and blood sugar, influencing genetic expression, and affecting brain chemical production.

Our gut microbiome is influenced by our genetics, our environment, and the foods we eat. When the intestines contain the right balance of good and bad bacteria, our gut is in a state of *symbiosis.* An imbalance of the microbiome is referred to as *dysbiosis* and is a primary source of inflammation. The relationship between the gut and the brain is so strong that one of the most noticeable symptoms of dysbiosis is fatigue.

The microbiome directly interacts with your gut's immune system. Remember, the brain and gut have a bidirectional relationship. These messages influence the brain's response to stress, brain hormone production, the activation of the brain's immune system, and the growth of new brain cells.[2] An imbalanced microbiome creates the right environment for intestinal permeability, which can cause inflammation and affect brain hormone production, which leads to depression, anxiety, cognitive dysfunction, and impaired social function.[3] It increases inflammation throughout the brain and the body, which then increases our risk for Alzheimer's, anxiety, memory loss, brain fog, and mood swings.

THE ROLE OF GLUTEN

All of this is especially important to know for the millions of sufferers that carry the risk genes for Celiac disease (CD) or gluten sensitivity. Both of these are considered to be autoimmune gastrointestinal and systemic immune disorders. They are characterized by inflammation and tissue remodeling in the small intestine. The disorder has a multifactorial etiology in which the triggering environmental factor—the gluten—and the main genetic factors, Human Leukocyte Antigen (HLA) at the DQA1*05 and DQB1*02 loci are well known, though less so DQB.

Sufferers experience an immune sensitivity to gliadin, a component of gluten, and its related proteins that are present in wheat, rye, barley, and to a lesser extent in other grains. The gliadin seizes control of their nervous system, unless they avoid these foods completely. The disease is characterized by a range of neurologic deficits, including peripheral neuropathy, dysautonomia, cerebellar ataxia, and encephalopathy. Gluten damages and inflames the microvilli. At the same time, the integrity of the gut wall is compromised, causing intestinal permeability, resulting in diarrhea, weight loss, constipation, and/or cramping. The presence of gut inflammation in Celiac appears to increase the chatter between bacteria and the immune system, leading to the release of bacterial products. For children under 2 years of age, these symptoms accompany a lack of weight gain and are often described as "failure to thrive."

Extended gluten exposure may affect the brain by disrupting the blood–brain barrier, which can cause symptoms in all three areas of the nervous system. CNS involvement is characterized by symptoms including headache; disabling brain fog; imbalance and incoordination; neuropsychiatric illness; mood, anxiety, eating, attention deficit, and autism spectrum disorders; and intellectual impairments. In one study of adult patients with Celiac, two-thirds had CNS complaints.[4] ANS involvement can manifest as orthostatic hypotension, postural orthostatic tachycardia, and autonomic neuropathy with uncompensated orthostatic hypotension due to lack of reflex heart rate acceleration. PNS involvement can lead to sensorimotor polyneuropathy and painful small fiber neuropathy. Celiac disease prevalence is increased for those with a positive family history of Celiac, other autoimmune diseases, IgA, type 1 diabetes, and Hashimoto's thyroiditis.

DIAGNOSING CELIAC DISEASE AND GLUTEN SENSITIVITY

The clinical presentation of gluten sensitivity varies from patient to patient. Genetic predisposition plays a key role in disease prevalence, and considerable progress has been made recently in identifying genes that are involved. About 90 to 95 percent of Celiac patients carry the genetic predisposition for gluten sensitivity, encoded by DQA1*05 and DQB1*02 alleles, compared to 10 percent of normal individuals in the general population, while only 30% of true cases and an equal percentage of normal individuals associate with DQ8.

While the genetic test gives a prediction of the susceptibility of developing CD, blood studies can give a clue to the presence of active allergic exposure by detecting IgA and IgG antibodies to endomysium, tissue transglutaminase, and gliadin. However, lacking these antibodies does not exclude the diagnosis, because when someone with Celiac has probably been following a gluten-free diet (GFD) or has immune incompetence, they may fail to display the appropriate immune response despite battling a gluten allergy.

The gold standard for identifying and diagnosing the disorder is endoscopic biopsy. Through this test, doctors can determine the relative health of the microvilli along with any inflammation and can determine the integrity of the intestinal endothelium. Yet even this type of testing can also produce false negatives and sampling errors.

Even if all of these tests return negative, you may have a non-Celiac gluten sensitivity. You may find that you feel and think better when you avoid gluten-filled foods like bread, pasta, pizza, and beer. In fact, the autoimmune or allergic symptoms that bring most people to medical attention feel better when they follow a stringent GFD, with or without the proper diagnosis. This is why a diagnosis of CD is confirmed if at least four of the following five criteria are fulfilled:

1. Typical symptoms of Celiac disease
2. Positivity of serum Celiac IgA class autoantibodies at high titer

3. HLA-DQ2 and/or HLA-DQ8 genotypes
4. Celiac enteropathy found on small bowel biopsy
5. Improvement following the adoption of a GFD

Celiac patients without any brain health symptoms may still show damage to the CNS. For instance, brain MRI may show a decrease in cortical and subcortical gray-matter volumes compared to controls. Frequently there is a loss of cerebellar volume and white matter abnormalities with conspicuous metabolic changes on PET indicative of inherent metabolic alterations in brain tissue function. Nuclear medicine single photon emission tomography (SPECT) imaging may suggest disruption of the BBB by revealing areas of decreased or increased regional brain perfusion. The highest incidence of white matter changes in Celiac cases occur in those complaining of headaches, especially migraines. A stunning majority of such cases show white matter changes in frontal brain regions, where executive function resides. In a small cohort of adult Celiac cases, all of whom had CNS complaints, all had evident abnormalities in regional cerebral blood flow on brain SPECT,[5] as well as, areas of regional cortical hypoperfusion. I have used brain PET/MRI in my patients with CD, and encountered widespread hypometabolism in cortical and cerebellar regions of the brain.

A Swedish biopsy registry of individuals with CD showed a moderately increased risk of depression and suicide when there was evidence of active inflammation in mucosal biopsies indicating active local and systemic autoimmunity.[6] There was a markedly increased risk of autism spectrum disorder in Celiac individuals with normal mucosa and a positive Celiac result in a blood test.[7]

TREATING CELIAC DISEASE WITH A GLUTEN-FREE DIET

The road to recovery starts with taking personal charge, acting like a detective, being on the lookout for brain dysfunction resulting from gluten sensitivity and excessive carbohydrate and dietary sugar ingestion. So states neurologist Dr. David Perlmutter, who believes as I do that treatment needs to be focused first on removing gluten from the diet while incorporating healthy fats to reduce body and brain inflammation, as we discussed in chapter 5.

Optimal brain and body health can only truly be restored by achieving one's ideal weight. Shifting your body's metabolism by going gluten-free is the first step in keeping you on-course for life-long changes in the way you relate to food.

Our diet modifies the microbiome, and the microbiome modifies our diet,[8] and ultimately our brain health. Remember the gut–brain axis: the gut contains more than 300 million neurons that monitor and inform the brain about our internal physiological and metabolic state.[9] So it's no surprise that the positive effect of brain health following a GFD has been reported in numerous cohort studies.[10] In adults, a positive response, defined as a significant reduction or resolution of headaches, varied from 50 percent to 100 percent in those who embarked on a GFD, and in children, the response rates ranged between 70 percent and 100 percent. A GFD can normalize the cortical hypoperfusion abnormalities. Although brain white matter changes are generally irreversible, patients on a strict GFD have a lower incidence of them.

Dietary analysis of patients with persistent symptoms, including headaches, show that up to 56 percent of patients consume traces of gluten even when they are strictly following a GFD. However, when they are even more careful, their symptoms improve.[11] You can test how well you are in compliance with an anti-gluten antigen monitor. These kits are commercially available, including a Wheat Gluten Elisa Kit to detect the total wheat protein/gluten in foods to avoid wheat allergy;[12] a hand-held gluten detector[13] marketed as Nima; and an interactive e-learning module that provides reliable gluten-free education.[14]

WATCH FOR FODMAPS

People with Celiac or non-Celiac gluten sensitivity may also find that their thinking and digestion are negatively impacted when they eat foods that fall into the FODMAP category. FODMAP stands for fermentable, oligo-, di-, mono-saccharides, and polyols. FODMAPs are a family of carbohydrates found in wheat and many other foods. FODMAPs are osmotic, which means they pull water into the intestinal tract, and so can cause fermentation in the intestinal tract when eaten in excess, possibly contributing to an imbalanced microbiome. The excess fermentation can cause bloating, gas, abdominal pain, diarrhea, and sometimes constipation.

According to Dr. Tom O'Bryan's book The Autoimmune Fix, if you currently suffer from abdominal complaints, you should consider removing the following FODMAPs from your diet:

- Almonds
- Apples
- Apricots
- Artichokes
- Asparagus
- Avocados
- Beets
- Blackberries
- Boysenberries
- Butternut squash
- Cabbage
- Cashews
- Cauliflower
- Celery
- Cherries
- Cranberries
- Currants
- Dates
- Figs
- Garlic
- Grapefruit
- Leeks
- Mangoes
- Mushrooms
- Nectarines
- Onions and shallots
- Peaches
- Pears
- Peas
- Persimmons
- Pistachios
- Plums
- Pomegranates
- Prunes
- Pumpkin
- Raisins
- Sugar snap peas
- Sweet potato and yams
- Watermelon

BOX 12.1

THERE IS MORE GLUTEN SENSITIVITY THAN EVER BEFORE

Celiac disease is an uncommon disease, amounting to only eight new cases per 100,000 persons annually in the United States, and no more than 0.17 percent of the population at any given time. Yet there has been an increase in the reported incidence and prevalence of reported cases in the United States and around the world.[15] What's more, there is a noticeable increase in the popularity of empiric gluten-free dietary management of autoimmune disease in general with an estimated 100 million Americans consuming gluten-free products each year. Factors that predict better rates of nervous system resolution after the initiation of a strict GFD include a strong family history of Celiac and shorter durations of symptoms prior to the diagnosis, while cases with longer duration of symptoms are at greater risk of an altered gut-brain axis.[16] The latter cases should be considered for immune modulatory therapy.

IVIG TREATMENT FOR CELIAC DISEASE

When there is evidence of a progressive autoimmune nervous system or brain disorder such as the one associated with severe CD, diet control is often not enough. The immune system is still in high gear from decades of allergic stimulation. The next step is to consider immune-modulatory therapy to treat associated CNS and PNS involvement. IVIg, alone or in combination with plasma exchange to potentiate its effect, should be considered in managing refractory nervous system involvement due to an altered gut-brain axis. Patients with ANS involvement manifesting as orthostatic intolerance should be treated symptomatically with agents that support vital signs such as hydration, dietary salt, and pharmaceuticals that increase blood pressure, manage heart rate, and when needed, pressure stockings.

IVIg therapies can reset the immune system by downregulating T-cell and B-cell activation, interfering with complement protein activation, and usurping the inflammatory cascade, while restoring the integrity of normal antibody production. Subcutaneous Ig (SCIg) therapy can be employed in children with common variable immune deficiency (CVID) with underlying Ig deficiencies as supplemental or replacement therapy to prevent recurrent bacterial infections, and in others with intestinal disease who deplete their stores due to inflammation and intestinal permeability.

Meet Christopher

Christopher is a 14-year-old eighth grader who came to see me. His mother told me that he was a colicky infant and suffered from life-long hypotonia: poor muscle tone. He has been diagnosed with childhood asthma and attention deficit hyperactivity disorder. He suffered from chronic pain, weakness, and tremors, and was now experiencing migraine headaches, agitation, palpitations, and mood disturbance veering toward depression. He had recently fainted at school and was diagnosed with obstructive sleep apnea and hypothyroidism.

I ordered a new round of testing for Christopher. We found him to have demyelinating neuropathy in the legs and orthostatic intolerance: two clear signs of autoimmune disorders. I wasn't surprised because as we know, if one person suffers from one autoimmune disorder, like Christopher's asthma, it's likely that he would have others. Calf and thigh epidermal nerve fiber biopsy showed a reduction in small fiber density.

However, the bloodwork showed something that no one ever tested for. He was positive for the Celiac HLA DQ2 genotype at the DQA1*05 and DQB1*02 loci. PET/MRI of the brain showed abnormal hippocampal structure with signs of early sclerosis suggesting inflammatory damage. There were areas of hypometabolism in the medial temporal lobes and in the frontal lobe. Volumetric analysis showed low hippocampal volumes with loss of the normal architecture, along with decreased associated white matter volume, and asymmetry of the size of the fornix (a bundle of nerve fibers in the brain that acts as the major output tract of the hippocampus). Thus, there were signs of brain changes that must have been evolving over many years due to altered autoimmunity and inflammation despite a GFD.

With this combination of neuropathy, dysautonomia, and neurocognitive and neuropsychiatric findings and the HLA DQ2 genotype, it was clear to me that Celiac was affecting Christopher's nervous system, even though he was much like any other high school student. He is now following a strict GFD, and he is slowly stabilizing his brain health issues and staying in school. He is also receiving IVIg therapy as initial support to his maturing nervous system and immune system.

STRESS AFFECTS THE BRAIN AND THE GUT

Research has clearly shown[17] that stress disrupts the body homoeostasis and manifests symptoms such as anxiety, depression, or even headache. We also know that the gut's microbiome changes as a response to stress. Stress can cause an upset stomach, and digestive issues cause us to feel stressed.[18] Dysbiosis can also be caused by stress.[19] Here's how it works: The microbiome sends chemical messengers to the brain that instruct the hypothalamus how to respond to stress. The hypothalamus tells the pituitary gland which stressors are the priorities, and the pituitary gland then sends messages telling the organs what hormones to produce. If your gut's microbiome is out of balance, the anxiety you woke up with won't go away and might even increase while you work all day. If you don't have the support in your gut needed to keep your brain calm, the severity of the stress response is higher, maintaining and reinforcing the stress hormones. Luckily, the same lifestyle interventions that modulate stress, which we discussed in part II of this book, can also modulate the microbiota. What's more, as you strengthen your microbiome, your emotional resiliency increases.

Meet Lila

Lila was a 29-year-old CrossFit instructor who was diagnosed with lupus and suffered from back pain, headaches, incoordination, and weakness that was beginning to interfere with her job. She also had a life-long history of intestinal problems that she mostly brushed aside because they really weren't holding her back from day-to-day living. Lila was also experiencing forgetfulness and was worried that she was experiencing memory loss. Her headaches were so severe she had taken herself to the emergency room for treatment. There, doctors found that Lila had pleocytosis, an inflammation found in the cerebrospinal fluid (CSF). This is a problem because CSF is identical to the fluid that bathes the brain. They also believed that she might have multiple sclerosis because of her overall weakness.

When she came to me, I explained that this inflammation may be causing her cognitive issues. Yet her brain scan was actually normal. Her total spine MRI showed disc problems, but there was nothing in it that would suggest anything more. However, when we did look at the brain MRI very carefully, I could see diminished volume. For someone as young as Lila, this shouldn't be happening. The good news was that we could rule out multiple sclerosis, because she didn't have the demyelination in the brain.

I also ordered a lumbar puncture to check on her previous diagnosis of pleocytosis. This time, the CSF revealed a neurodegenerative process. The spinal tap showed a high protein ratio, which is a sure sign of a brain process that has been compromised and now leaking into the spinal fluid. This was causing the shrinkage in brain volume, which led to a brain that was not working as quickly as it's supposed to. This was the cause of Lila's memory issues. A PET/MRI showed that the only part of her brain that was working at capacity was the frontal lobes where executive functions work. The rest of the brain's poor functioning could not be connected to the spinal fluid problem.

We decided to reflect back on her health history. She told me about the intestinal problems she typically experienced, including both frequently occurring diarrhea and constipation. She also shared that her mother had the same complaints, so didn't pay much attention to Lila's digestive health. I decided to order bloodwork including Celiac genotyping that showed a positive HLA DQ2 genotype at the DQA1*05 and DQB1*02 loci. Because we know that Celiac can so aggressively affect brain health, I immediately put Lila on a strict GFD.

Today, Lila is doing much better. But when she came to see me a few months ago, she was perplexed. She could not understand why her Celiac was affecting her brain now, when the tests showed that she had it all along as part of her genetic makeup. I explained that she started having the neurological complaints when some of the other immunological things going on caused enough immune deterioration. Her immune system was finally attacking the brain causing a neurodegenerative process. However, I assured her that if she could maintain a GFD for the rest of her life, she would continue to be symptom-free when it came to her brain health.

13

Concussions Leave
Their Mark

Concussion, also known as mild traumatic brain injury (mTBI), is a common brain event that carries a high risk of neuropsychiatric manifestations for which treatment of the associated psychological disturbance is as important as addressing the injury itself. Once considered a part of post-concussive syndrome,[1] it is now known that mTBI can lead to anxiety, depression, and cognitive impairment.[2] What's more, people who have had concussions risk poor attention and alcohol and drug abuse.[3] Some individuals may linger into more protracted periods of healing with seizures and disabling headaches. These symptoms may last weeks, months, or up to a year after a single event, depending upon the severity of head injury. Second, third, and fourth episodes of repeated severe concussions, especially in a short period between events, may result in a proportionate length and severity of recovery and a heightened predisposition to permanent neurological or psychiatric deficits.

While not all blows or jolts to the head result in a concussion, those that do are typically associated with at least a brief change in mental status. The immediate and short-term symptoms associated with concussion reflect the direct blow to the brain that leads to a transient loss of function of the tissue underneath the head injury rather than primary functional cerebral disturbance or permanent structural damage.

Concussion leads to a systemic immune response to damaged neurons across a disrupted BBB.[4] The loss of the integrity of the BBB results in localized and

immediate damage to the affected portion of the brain with delayed effects at
a distance from the injury. This is due to immediate disturbance of brain functions depending upon the areas affected. If the injury occurred in the frontal
lobe, executive and motor functions would be affected; in the parietal lobe,
spatial and sensory integration would be compromised; in the temporal lobe, it
would affect memory and mood stability. Any such damage can also lead to a
combination of motor, cognitive, perceptive sensory, emotional, and psychosocial consequences that can be devastating and potentially long-lasting.

Any opening to the BBB exposes innate brain immune cells to antigens,
leading to the release of immunologic or biological markers across the BBB
from the brain into the systemic circulation and in the opposite direction
from the bloodstream into the cranial cavity.[5] These markers reflect the initial
insult as well as the evolution of a cascade of secondary damage. They have the
potential to not only signal and monitor the evolution of the injury process in
the systemic circulation and brain, but to limit the spread of damage through
the activation of brain receptors.

There is an experimental model of concussion that closely mirrors the
situation in humans and accounts for the alterations in mood and memory
that are commonly seen. Animals given a closed-head injury develop a disturbance in electrical connectivity between the hippocampus and the prefrontal
lobe, which comprises an important link in the human cortical-limbic circuit.[6]

Symptoms from concussion will range based on the time frame immediately after the incident. In the early stage of a concussion, meaning the first
minutes to hours after injury, symptoms include:

- Headache
- Dizziness or vertigo
- Lack of awareness or surroundings
- Nausea or vomiting

The late stage ranges from a few days following an incident to a few weeks.
Symptoms at this time can include:

- Persistent low-grade headache
- Lightheadedness
- Inattention and impaired concentration

- Memory disturbance
- Easy fatigability
- Irritability and low frustration tolerance
- Intolerance of bright lights
- Difficulty focusing vision
- Intolerance of loud noises and tinnitus

Post-concussive symptoms are seen in up to a third of cases and persist for up to several months after primary injury, tapering to about 2.5 percent at 1 year.[7] Pervasive symptoms of concussion lead to a disturbance in adaptive independent functioning. Children who sustain concussive head injury face different challenges than adults. Young children face increased vulnerability due to concomitant maturational periods of brain and neuropsychological development, whereas adolescents face greater demands on cognitive, organization, and problem-solving skills due to deficits in executive functioning. Educational issues that emerge later related to concussion may be inappropriately managed or incorrectly attributed to other factors.

IDENTIFYING CONCUSSION IS THE KEY FOR HEADING OFF A MENTAL HEALTH DISASTER

Although it is likely that younger children may recover better from a concussion than their older peers, recovery from an mTBI seems to depend on many factors, including injury features and environmental influences. Neural brain plasticity plays a role in the apparent relative resilience of younger brains and in protecting most children from the devastating effects of head trauma. Several factors that might mitigate the influence of injury (particularly for children) include access to mental health services and the support of people like parent caregivers and institutions like school systems. These findings corroborate the associations between repeated injuries, particularly sports-related concussion and dementia, psychiatric disorders, and even attempted suicide reported in the recent literature.[8] Investigators in Quebec[9] studied the risk of suicide in 135,703 children up to age 17 who sustained an mTBI, noting a higher risk of later depression.

Today we can employ sensitive neuroimaging studies such as PET/MRI with special volumetric analysis to investigate the damage to the brain stemming from a concussion, even years after the injury has occurred. We can also use biological markers in the blood, including the Banyan Trauma Indicator to help streamline the decision to proceed to brain scanning.[10] This is how we link pervasive neurological deficits, such as cognitive and neuropsychiatric complaints, including memory loss, intellectual impairments, anxiety, and depression to an original insult.

Severe or recurrent head injury potentially goes a step further, resulting in distinctive pathological changes in the brain reminiscent of a neurodegenerative disorder due to the deposition of tau proteins. When seen microscopically in a biopsy or postmortem tissue specimen of a patient with neurocognitive and neuropsychiatric complaints, they tell the story of the irreversible brain damage seen in cases of chronic traumatic encephalopathy.[11]

Meet Sarah

Sarah came into my office when she was a 23-year-old college student. She told me that she had severe migraines for a few years beginning at age 4, which she was told might have been related to a chickenpox vaccine. When she was 6, she was in a sledding accident, striking her head and sustaining a black eye.

By the time Sarah was 7, the migraines diminished, and she tested into a gifted students program. At age 9, she sustained a second concussion during gymnastics practice, and that same summer returned from a family vacation in rural Virginia with a tick bite behind her ear. She was then tested for Lyme disease, but the results were negative. However, she developed left knee pain later that year and a rash, prompting intravenous antibiotics for a month with improvement.

Sarah played field hockey and lacrosse in middle school and high school, only suffering minor injuries. When she was 14, the migraines returned, and she tested positive for Lyme and took the oral antibiotics that were standard of care to treat it. However, she was now struggling with extreme fatigue, leading her to take a gap year from high school before starting college.

At age 19, in her first year of college, there were more frequent seizures, once awakening her from a deep sleep whereupon she rose quickly out of bed and fell, striking her head on a metal doorstop. That year she had a severe flu reaction to the meningitis vaccine. The next year she went back to school part-time with academic accommodations. At age 21, she was still at school and had a seizure after a late night shower falling slowly to the ground, hitting her head on the tile floor. Afterward she had trouble concentrating, weak legs, shakiness, and depression.

When I saw her in the fall of 2017, she was stressed over school, unable to concentrate with weakness, lightheadedness, and imbalance. She complained of headaches. Electrodiagnostic studies showed mild distal demy-elinating and axonal polyneuropathy, and thinning of the parietal cortex with hypometabolism presumably in the area of recurrent head injury on PET/MRI. The reductions in the hippocampal volumes explained her propensity for seizures and mood and cognitive impairments, and suggested the need to screen her for post-infectious (I-Cubed) and autoantibody-associated autoimmunity. In fact, a low titer GAD65 antibody and reactive Lyme serology were both found in the blood. However it was uncertain whether the Lyme was active or she was experiencing persistent nervous system symptoms of post-treatment Lyme disease syndrome (PTLDS). That label postulates the presence of non-viable spirochetes or their remnants that elicit a positive serologic response.

Sarah was started on IVIg and encouraged to drink plenty of fluids, ingest salt, and slowly return to school. One year later she was stable, back at school, and had not had further head injury, infection, seizures, or other sources of immunologic stimulation. However, a year into school, she felt like she had worsened due to recurrent fatigue and cognitive and mood disturbances. A repeat PET/MRI showed further progression of cortical hypometabolism extending to both temporal lobes and hippocampi reminiscent of autoimmune encephalopathy.[12] A lumbar puncture showed reactive Lyme serology in the blood and cerebrospinal fluid (CSF) with negative IgG and IgM Western blots and a normal Lyme Index (that measures the ratio of Borrelia-specific antibodies in the CSF and serum) confirming the absence of active neurological Lyme, and instead suggesting PTLDS.[13]

A key to understanding Sarah's worsening brain illness lies partly in I-Cubed, and in the sequela of concussion. Research suggests heightened cortical immunity long after a standard course of antibiotics for Lyme disease;[14] and a greater risk for autoimmune encephalopathy after an mTBI, presumably by allowing passage of circulatory cytokines, autoantibodies, and other mitigating substances across a disrupted BBB.[15] For the present time, Sarah is being monitored closely on antibiotics and IVIg therapy. Physicians faced with similar patients must decide the appropriate use of antibiotics, IVIg, and biological therapies such as rituximab, alone or in combination, to treat post-infectious and autoantibody-associated brain illness in the setting of prior mTBIs.

TREATING CONCUSSIONS

Contrary to conventional wisdom, medically prescribed excessive cognitive and physical rest contributes to delayed recovery, making supervised and graduated physical activity, and the introduction of cognitive behavioral therapy (CBT)[16,17] to reduce cognitive biases and misattribution as effective means of enhancing recovery.

With proper identification of concussions and the autoimmune response they trigger, sufferers of head injury may utilize the right therapies and limit both short- and long-term damage. Selective serotonin and norepinephrine reuptake inhibitors (SSRIs and SNRIs) antidepressants contribute to hippocampal neurogenesis by increasing neuronal signaling along cortical-limbic pathways prone to injury by head trauma,[18] suggesting that they offer an effective therapy for both depression and mTBI recovery because of their favorable action upon the injured neuronal circuits that produce cortical hypometabolism seen on PET/MRI.

Returning to exercise should be carried out only under medical supervision, but should not be inordinately delayed due to a fear of subsequent injury. As I started earlier, the reintroduction of physical activity appears to improve brain function and hastens recovery.

Meet Matthew

Except for mild obsessive-compulsive disorder and motor tics, Matthew was a completely normal rising sophomore attending a prominent northeast college. He was working as group leader at a day camp in the summer of 2017 when he was hit in the head with a basketball during recreational play. For a moment he was dazed and noticed that he had a headache, but the camp nurse said he was fine and to return to work. Later that day he participated in a counselor's diving contest whereupon he felt an "explosion" in his head when he went underwater.

For the rest of the summer he was unable to work, and he relaxed at home but could not read, watch television, or look at his phone or computer screen because of headaches. A local psychologist diagnosed him with post-concussive syndrome and suggested that Matthew should not return to school in the fall. Alone at home, away from friends, and in pain, he became increasingly lonely and angry. At the same time, he was troubled by brain fog, sleep disturbances, intrusive thoughts, and a progressive inability to talk. He avoided his friends as he was embarrassed about his situation, but he exercised by walking laps around the house and at his local high school track.

A psychiatrist diagnosed him with PTSD and prescribed anti-anxiety medication. When he developed delusional fears of getting additional concussions, his family knew that his brain was not healing. At this point they took him to another psychiatrist who diagnosed severe depression. He was placed on fluoxetine and aripiprazole and started CBT with neurorehabilitation and supervised exercise. Within a month on this medication and cognitive behavioral therapy, he experienced a remarkable reawakening of his brain, with complete dissipation of headaches and a return to normal thinking. Two years after the incident, he was able to return to college.

One of the reasons why Matthew was able to respond so quickly to pharmacotherapy and CBT lies in the ability of the hippocampus to repair through neural plasticity especially under the action of selective serotonin anti-depressants. I refer to the hippocampus as the "shock absorber" of the brain because of its vulnerability, and endowment with an enormous capacity to engage in neurogenesis through its innate stem cells. Stress and depression reduces neurogenesis; however stimulating serotonergic transmission promotes neurogenesis in hippocampal circuits and in other affected brain areas. Matthew's isolation initially led to poor results, but once he was instructed to leave the dark room, and actively and wisely reha-bilitated, he was able to foster the innate neural plasticity and regenerative powers of his brain.

14

Neuroendocrine and Mast Cell Activity Determine How You Respond to Stress

Stress is a normal physiological response that is initiated any time we are faced with adversity in our environment; the way we process stress, and the way our body responds to it, influences our resiliency and the way we deal with and overcome these challenges. One type of adversity is living with chronic diseases. As we know, on their own they disrupt our quality of life and day-to-day life activities, and that, in and of itself, can lead to psychological stress. What's more, the stress response can instigate the onset and progression of pain, cognitive disorder, and psychiatric disorders. In short, stress induces diseases, which can exacerbate the stress severity, resulting in a vicious cycle.[1]

Stress due to chronic diseases, dementia, brain trauma, poor sleep habits, immobilization, isolation, noise, high workload, unstable job, annoying work environment, and other modern life conditions all contribute to unwanted changes in the CNS. These changes include cognitive disorders that are caused by the resulting inflammation, altered secretion of growth factors, production of pro-inflammatory cytokines, and increased oxidative stress that disrupts the BBB and affect brain volume.[2,3]

Stress can also induce the changes in the peripheral and autonomic nervous systems, affecting immune cells throughout the body, notably mast cells. Mast cells are a type of immune cells found throughout the body that are important actors in normal immunity and serve specialized defense responses against parasites and other infectious pathogens. Mast cells can also combat allergic reactions. However, when activated as a result of stress, they can cause BBB disruption, neuroinflammation, and neurodegeneration.[4,5,6,7] The number, distribution, and activation status of mast cells in the brain is not constant, but varies due to one's environment, behavioral changes, and physiological state. Mast cells migrate from the blood into various tissues where they mature and acquire specific characteristics influenced by their environment. A change in your emotional state and the way you handle stress may be the first clue to a neuroendocrine dysfunction that, left untreated, can be associated with permanent neural injury and potentially life-threatening consequences.

As we've discussed, the hypothalamic-pituitary-adrenal (HPA) axis is where the brain becomes the director of the pituitary gland and its neural and endocrine, or *neuroendocrine*, ties to the body as a whole. The hypothalamus is the area of the brain that secretes the chemical factors that make up a variety of hormones that get secreted into the bloodstream. These hormones influence the pituitary gland, which in turn influences other organs in the body, particularly the adrenal gland, by its own stimulating hormones. The HPA axis regulates the release of the hormones epinephrine, norepinephrine, and cortisol, released by the adrenal gland; stimulates bone growth and thyroid gland hormone production; and controls the sex hormones that influence the menstrual cycle and readiness of the ovaries and uterus for pregnancy and childbirth, and the maintenance of male hormone levels. When the HPA axis is affected by the immune system, illness, or infection, or by inadvertent stress, there can be deficient blood pressure and pulse management in addition to neurocognitive and intellectual decline.

The initial stress response protects the body; however, chronic stress and chronic pain can be an underlying cause of many health problems. The reason is that stress and the immune system interact bidirectionally, enhancing the stress response.[8] At the same time, stressful conditions can inhibit the immune response, causing inflammatory conditions including neuroinflammation.[9,10] When infections in the CNS cross the BBB, they can take up residence in the brain. There, they secrete a full range of cytokines and other inflammatory mediators that stimulate activity in the HPA axis. A change in blood pressure, heart rate, sweating, temperature regulation, hair growth, and other autonomic nervous system functions may be the first clue to neuroendocrine disorders. Unrecognized and untreated, there may be potentially disastrous consequences ranging from mental changes to permanent neural injury. For instance, dysautonomia, a balance impairment combined with low blood pressure, is a common feature of post-infectious nervous system autoimmunity. Another condition, postural orthostatic tachycardia, presents with accelerated heart rate upon tilting or standing, but without hypotension. Orthostatic hypotension leads to an abrupt fall in systolic blood pressure upon standing or tilting.

Chronic fatigue is another common phenomenon that occurs during inflammatory and autoimmune conditions. Although pain and psychological factors may influence fatigue, there is an increasing understanding that there is a genetic basis and that activation of the immune system itself is an essential generator of fatigue.[11] Fatigue is generated at least partly through innate immunity responses, and mast cells are strong activators of the disturbed immunity. It is therefore to be expected that fatigue is a significant complaint among patients with mast cell disorders.

MAST CELL ACTIVATION SYNDROME

Mast cells, also known as mastocytes, are cells that reside in the connective tissue surrounding the joints. They contain granules rich in histamine and heparin, which are immune system triggers. When activated, they release granules that play a role in mounting an inflammatory allergic response, contributing to the body's defense against infectious intruders. For instance, mast cells are released in the setting of allergic, post-infectious, autoimmune, and inflammatory states typified by high levels of circulating cytokines.

Mast cell activation syndrome (MCAS) occurs when patients have frequent and inappropriate episodes of mast cell activation, which typically looks like an allergic reaction even when there is no allergen present. Certain mutations in mast cells can produce populations of identical mast cells—called clones—that overproduce and spontaneously activate. These abnormal cells can grow uncontrollably and are unusually sensitive to activation.

MCAS responds well to antihistamine medications. A rapid onset is associated with anaphylaxis, abrupt wheezing, hypotension, tachycardia, nausea, vomiting, abdominal cramping, and diarrhea; a slower release of mast cells is associated with flushing and nasal stuffiness.

The symptoms vary widely from person to person and are often episodic and wax and wane with varying degrees of intensity, sometimes worsening over time, making it difficult to properly diagnose. For instance, in a cohort of 413 patients with MCAS,[12] a history of frequent drug reactions was noted in 23 percent, chronic abdominal pain in 22 percent, chronic depression in 16 percent, frequent environmental allergies in 19 percent, recurrent pharyngitis or tonsillitis in 14 percent, osteoarthritis or obesity in 13 percent, chronic anxiety and panic attacks in 12 percent, fainting due to hypotension in 11 percent, and postural orthostatic tachycardia syndrome in 10 percent. On physical examination, 47 percent appeared tired; 42 percent looked chronically ill; 39 percent looked swollen, puffy, or inflamed; 37 percent were obese; 34 percent had rashes; 28 percent were tachycardic; 12 percent had cognitive dysfunction; 12 percent were physically weak; and 11 percent were anxious or depressed.

HASHIMOTO THYROIDITIS AND ENCEPHALOPATHY: TWO INTRIGUING DISORDERS

Hashimoto thyroiditis (HT), the most common neuroendocrine disorder that affects the thyroid gland, rarely develops into a full-fledged autoimmune encephalopathy, which is associated with the action of high titers of circulating antibodies that permeate the BBB, targeting higher intellectual areas.[13] However, it can occur, and neurologists have been pursuing the association for over 50 years. In 1966, British neurologists[14] first described Hashimoto encephalopathy (HE) in a 40-year-old man who had epileptic and stroke-like episodes of confusion and agitation 1 year following a diagnosis of hypothyroidism. Researchers Jellinek and Ball[15] later studied the same patient who died at the age of 62. An autopsy showed no remaining thyroid tissue and cerebrovascular changes. The authors postulated an autoimmune disturbance as the cause of thyroiditis and encephalopathy. Since then, the diagnosis of HE rests upon the presence of thyroiditis, with measurably high titers of thyroid peroxidase or thyroglobulin antibodies, clinical encephalopathy (as evidenced by clouding of consciousness with reduced wakefulness, attention, or cognitive function), and absent evidence of an active CNS infection. However, it is unknown how or whether antithyroid antibodies and thyroid dysfunction contribute to the pathogenesis of encephalopathy. Although principally neurological in presentation, there can be telltale signs of most thyroid diseases, such as weight gain and constant fatigue.

Meet Danny

At age 17, my patient Danny complained of an emerging depression and sense of isolation. His mother, Ivy, was at her wit's end. Danny had gained 100 pounds in just 6 months: a tremendous amount for a young man. He simply couldn't get out of bed, was constantly irritable, and battled with a loss of stamina, headaches, and memory loss. Throughout his teen years, Danny had suffered from numerous head traumas. He had received several concussions playing high school basketball, and earlier in his life, he was bullied at school and punched in the head. Ivy took Danny to every major medical institution in New York City. As a very avid researcher, she came to me only after she had exhausted all of her other resources. As Danny told me, "I've seen 50,000 doctors, and I hate coming to the doctor."

When they walked into my office, Ivy already thought she knew what was troubling Danny, because her doctors had told her that her son's head injuries were causing his depression. Yet she didn't quite trust the findings. Ivy was right. As soon as I examined Danny, I knew that the head trauma wasn't the only problem, because his neurologic symptoms could not account for his weight gain. Instead, I wondered if there was an autoimmune component. Something else had to have preceded the head injuries that triggered an autoimmune response.

After taking the appropriate blood testing, I found that Danny did in fact have several autoimmune issues in addition to involvement of all three areas of the nervous system: CNS, PNS, and ANS. His pituitary gland was malfunctioning and there were low levels of testosterone and other important hormones. He had low cortisol levels, which showed that his adrenal gland wasn't functioning well. His thyroid gland was enlarged with elevated titers of thyroid peroxidase (TPO) and antithyroglobulin antibodies (ATA), signifying HT, which was later proven on a fine needle aspiration of the gland. These, along with his unexplained weight gain, were all sure signs that Danny was suffering from a neuroendocrine pituitary disorder.

I ordered a further round of testing. First, Danny had a brain PET/MRI that showed a lesion in the tail of the left hippocampus tail and areas of hypometabolism in both temporal and parietal lobes of the brain. In addition, a brain SPECT showed hypoperfusion deficits in both temporal and the right parietal lobes related to disruption of the BBB, in the same areas that were hypometabolic. This was very significant and likely to reflect initial BBB disruption leading to brain tissue changes. Serum and cerebrospinal fluid testing showed that he did not have Lyme disease.

The treatment goal was to get Danny back to school so that he could finish high school. Treatment began with weekly intravenous immunoglobulin, which was later combined with a tapering course of alternate day prednisone to treat presumptive Hashimoto's encephalopathy (HE), leading to significant improvement.

Leaders in the field propose categorizing cases of HE as a form of AE after exclusion of other syndromes associated with well-defined autoantibodies.[16] The relatively few biopsy and postmortem examinations available in patients with pathogenic serum antibodies have shown infiltrating inflammatory T-cells with cytotoxic granules in close apposition to hippocampal neurons, analogous to microscopic vasculitis.[17]

Ivy wanted to address Danny's weight gain, and we discussed that neither caloric restriction nor hormone balancing were the solutions. Instead, we would begin by addressing the immune system with the right medications supplemented by the diet featured in this book, in the hopes that his hormone levels would rebalance once the pituitary gland and hypothalamus were functioning again. Danny now has hope that he will feel better, has increased energy, and has a plan to return to high school in the fall.

I couldn't forget about the concussions Danny suffered and what role they might have played in his illness. The mechanisms underlying TBI and AE are both associated with BBB disruption. They also result in the triggering of immunological factors that promoted neuronal inflammation and degeneration.[18] Overlapping abnormalities on SPECT and PET/MRI in Danny's case suggested that BBB disruption caused by these earlier concussions might have placed him at greater risk for developing HE or the equivalent of a reversible AE, by allowing the passage of circulatory cytokines, autoantibodies, and other mitigating substances across a disrupted BBB.

DIABETES MELLITUS: NAVIGATING THE MECHANISMS OF AUTOIMMUNITY

Both type I and type II diabetes (T1D and T2D) are neuroendocrine disorders that are associated with diverse metabolic processes that stem from hyperglycemia due to deficient secretion or action of insulin. Typically, diabetes patients are also at risk for developing secondary kidney, vascular, neurological, and ophthalmologic complications. Those affecting the brain and optic nerve are of particular importance because they may lead to permanent and disabling deficits that affect normal nervous system functioning.

T1D usually develops before the age of 30, whereas T2D patients are typically older, often obese, and at high risk for high cholesterol and heart disease. In the United States alone, more than one million people are living with the more severe type, T1D, with approximately 80 people per day or

30,000 individuals per year newly diagnosed. The global incidence of T1D is increasing at a rate of approximately 3 percent to 4 percent per year, notably among younger children.

In the past several years, research suggests the importance of genetic, environmental, infectious, and inflammatory mechanisms as the underlying causes of T1D. First, T1D appears to be caused by autoimmune mechanisms directed against the insulin-producing β-cells. Studies have shown that up to 90 percent of T1D patients test positive for autoantibodies. The pancreas of all newly diagnosed T1D patients show inflammation in the region of β-cells. The autopsies of children who die prematurely with T1D show pancreatic islet cell membrane-bound superantigens, indicating integrated bacterial or viral genes. One other possible mechanism of infection-induced autoimmunity of insulin-producing β-cells in the pancreas occurs through bystander activation, whereby the infection of neighboring β-cells stimulates local inflammation with the appearance of T-cells and other inflammatory cells that release inflammatory proteins that lead to killing of β-cells.

T1D occurs with increased frequency in association with several other autoimmune and neuroendocrine disorders, including Graves' disease, pernicious anemia, HT, myasthenia gravis, antiphospholipid antibody syndrome, and Addison disease. The gut's microbiome may also play a role. While it is less diverse and protective in normal individuals, it is now thought that those with T1D may have disturbed their microbiome in their early development, predisposing them to T1D. As we learned, an unbalanced microbiome can negatively influence the body's immunity, favoring increased intestinal permeability and therefore the establishment of harmful autoimmunity.

Viruses, with their potential to induce immune responses and inflammation, have been suspected of initiating an autoimmune process. Some microbial and host proteins can actually resemble their host cell organs and may go unrecognized by the immune system. This mechanism is known as molecular mimicry.

NEW WAYS FOR TREATING DIABETES

Insulin replacement has been the primary treatment of all forms of diabetes for almost a century, but inadequate control of its delivery has allowed a number of complications to markedly diminish the quality of life of affected individuals. The recognition that a subset of patients presents an autoimmune form of T1D is now well accepted and has led to different approaches to therapy. The spontaneous but temporary remission after onset of T1D, known as the honeymoon period, reflecting reduced stress on residual β-cells after initial insulin treatment, appears to be the window of opportunity to exploit the use of different therapies such as IVIg to block the autoimmune response, early in the course of the disease before appearance of hyperglycemia, and while there are sufficient β cells remaining.

Porphyria

A Misdiagnosed Neurogenetic Disorder

Porphyria is a rare neurologic disorder that causes a predisposition to drug sensitivity. It occurs in individuals of all racial and ethnic backgrounds, although it is rarely reported in the African American community. Women are affected by symptomatic porphyria more often than men, and it is most often diagnosed in women in their 20s or 30s, but may occur at or just after puberty. Onset before puberty is extremely rare.

Porphyrins are the main precursors of heme, an essential constituent that is found in different mechanisms of the body. It is found in hemoglobin, which transports oxygen in the blood; myoglobin, and in muscle cells where it stores oxygen molecules. Heme is also a component of the liver enzyme P450, which metabolize a variety of drugs in the body, especially antibiotics. Mutations in the genes for enzymes in the porphyrin pathways lead to insufficient production of heme and consequently a reduced level of oxygen in the blood, liver, and muscle cells. The result is an accumulation of porphyrins, which in high concentration are toxic to the body.

One common form of porphyria, called acute intermittent porphyria (AIP), occurs when there is a mutation in the hydroxymethylbilane synthase (*HMBS*) gene, which encodes the enzyme porphobilinogen deaminase (PBGD) that is crucial to the heme biosynthetic pathway. A person who has porphyria will seek medical attention when they take an excessive or prolonged courses of sulfa antibiotics, or one of the many other drugs toxic to porphyrin synthesis. Drugs that are toxic to porphyrin metabolism also impair the P450 system of the liver. Worse, when liver function declines, the body loses its ability to clear the drug from blood circulation, leading to more porphyrin toxicity. When this happens, less oxygen is available to the muscles and red blood cells, leading to body-wide crisis.

A diagnosis of porphyria can be difficult because the symptoms are not specific to the disorder, and they can come and go. The symptoms associated with various forms of porphyria differ. It is important to note that people who have one type of porphyria do not develop any of the other types. Porphyria is classified into two groups: "hepatic" (liver) and "erythropoietin" (blood-forming) types. Either can be associated with a range of symptoms and physical findings that can potentially involve multiple organ systems of the body.

Abdominal pain, which is usually severe, is the most common symptom associated with acute porphyria and often the initial sign of an attack. This pain is typically steady and widespread. Less often, abdominal pain is described as cramping. Pain may also occur in the neck, lower back, buttocks, or arms and legs. Gastrointestinal symptoms are also common and can include nausea, vomiting, constipation or diarrhea, and abdominal swelling and bloating. Urinary retention can also occur, along with dark or reddish urine. Abnormally low sodium levels (hyponatremia) may develop rapidly during an attack and contribute to the onset of seizures. People with porphyria are also extremely pale and particularly sensitive to sun exposure.

Neurological symptoms often accompany porphyria indicating damage to all categories of the nervous system: CNS, PNS, and ANS.

Among patients with AIP, 20 percent to 58 percent have CNS neuropsychiatric symptoms during acute exacerbations.[1] Psychiatric manifestations include hysteria, anxiety, depression, phobias, psychosis, agitation, delirium, and restlessness.[2] Some patients develop psychosis similar to schizophrenia. Other CNS neurological manifestations include seizures. The associated PNS involvement presents as a peripheral neuropathy with symptoms of numbness, tingling, or burning sensations that usually begin in the feet and hands. Affected individuals may develop muscle weakness in the legs that may progress to affect the arms and the trunk of the body, eventually causing loss or impairment of motor function. They may experience an ascending paralysis, which manifests itself typically over a month. Sufferers may first develop numbness and tingling in their feet, then they get so weak that they can end up in a wheelchair, temporarily. Once the episode is over, they typically get somewhat better and they recover.

Involvement of the ANS typically includes debilitating hypotension and reflex tachycardia upon standing or with exercising. Attacks of AIP typically develop over several hours, however affected individuals usually recover from an attack within days. If an acute attack is not diagnosed or promptly treated, recovery can take weeks or longer. Most affected individuals do not exhibit any symptoms in between episodes. Neurological involvement occurs in a stepwise manner worsening with each attack and overshadowed by the systemic manifestations. Failure to recognize porphyria as the cause of an attack can lead to the erroneous diagnosis of a kidney and bladder infection or acute appendicitis, with unnecessary diagnostic procedures or empiric antibiotics. Such medications, when toxic to the p450 enzyme system of the liver, can then create a vicious circle aggravating the severity, frequency, and length of attacks, and increasing the risk of nervous system damage.

A prospective study of the molecular epidemiology of gene defects among individuals with AIP[3] showed that there are as many as 78 different disease-causing mutations. Two of the reported patients in that study demonstrated paralysis resembling Guillain-Barre syndrome. Their nerves showed segmental demyelination, cellular inflammation, and degeneration of nerve fibers in cutaneous nerve biopsy tissues. In rare cases, the muscles used to breathe can become involved and potentially cause life-threatening respiratory failure. Some individuals develop psychological symptoms including irritability, depression, anxiety, insomnia, hallucinations, paranoia, disorientation, and altered consciousness ranging from excessive drowsiness to agitation.

Symptoms usually occur as episodes or "attacks" that develop over the course of several hours or a few days, and resolve within days. However, if an acute attack is not diagnosed and treated promptly, recovery can take much longer, ranging from weeks or months. Most affected individuals do not exhibit any symptoms in between episodes. The course and severity of attacks are highly variable from one person to another. Attacks are much more common in women than men, probably because of menstrual cycle hormones. Approximately 3 percent to 5 percent of affected individuals, predominantly women, experience recurrent attacks, which are defined as more than four per year, for a period of many years. Although symptoms usually resolve after an attack, some individuals may develop chronic pain. Nerve damage and associated muscle weakness from a severe attack improves over time, but such improvement may take many months to resolve fully.

The typical person suffering from porphyria experiences acute attacks of abdominal pain, which are often misdiagnosed as kidney stones, urinary tract infection, or appendicitis. Sufferers may be dismissed by their doctors as "crazy" because their symptoms may seem unfounded. To make matters more complicated, individuals with porphyria often have neuropsychiatric symptoms, like depression. Typically, their frequent stomach pain brings them to the doctor, who upon examination cannot find the cause of their complaints and sends them off with antidepressants or antibiotics in an attempt to assuage them. Unfortunately, these people are very likely to have allergic reactions to one or more of the medications.

Many drugs that are used to treat common neurological disorders can also provoke an attack of porphyria, including:

- Sulfa-based antibiotics and antifungal agents fluconazole and ketoconazole
- Ergotamine alkaloid drugs, including Cafergot, used to treat migraines

BOX 15.1

FOR MORE INFORMATION

The American Porphyria Foundation's website, https://porphyria foundation.org, is a wonderful resource if you think you may be suffering from this condition. It features a comprehensive database of drugs known to incite an attack.

- Anticonvulsants such as carbamazepine, phenytoin, and valproate used in seizure management
- Pain medications like oxycodone and ketamine

PORPHYRIA'S GENETIC COMPONENT

Porphyria is a multifactorial disorder, which means that genetic, systemic, and environmental factors must occur in combination in order for someone to develop symptoms. Individuals with porphyria have a mutation in the *HMBS* gene, causing the protein component of the gene to be either faulty, inefficient, or absent. Depending upon the functions of the particular protein, this can affect many organ systems of the body.

The majority of people with this genetic mutation do not necessarily develop symptoms of porphyria without additional factors, or *triggers*. These factors may not be the same for every individual, and susceptibility to specific triggers may vary during a patient's lifetime. Established triggers for AIP attack include infections, alcohol, smoking, hormonal factors, and physical or mental stress, beyond the known medications affecting heme synthesis.[4] Most of these triggers are believed to stimulate heme production in the liver. The *HMBS* gene then creates or encodes the enzyme PBGD, which is necessary for the process of heme biosynthesis. Mutations in the *HMBS* gene lead to deficient levels of PBGD in the body, which in turn can lead to the accumulation and release of the porphyrin precursors, delta5-aminolevulinic acid (delta-ALA) and PBG from the liver.

Low-grade inflammation may play a role in porphyria and affect the nervous system by altering the BBB. Just as injury causes a systemic inflammatory response syndrome, and microbial pathogen-associated molecular patterns activate innate immature immune cells through the process of pattern recognition receptors,[5] metabolic injury in AIP is thought to the release endogenous "damage"-associated molecular patterns that activate innate immunity. Excessive deposition of heme and porphyrins are reported to activate the complement system,[6] and patients with symptomatic AIP who develop malnutrition or hepatic inflammation at the height of their illness will have higher levels of systemic inflammation.[7]

TESTING AND TREATING PORPHYRIA

There are laboratory tests that can identify elevated levels of porphyrins excreted in the urine and stool, and whether the levels of the principal enzymes that causes the deficient synthesis is reduced. Screening tests to measure the levels of the PBG in urine are essential to confirm a diagnosis of porphyria. Acute attacks are always accompanied by increased excretion of PBG.

Molecular genetic testing is not essential to confirm the diagnosis because the porphyrin biochemical findings are characteristic. However, molecular genetic testing to detect a mutation in the *HMBS* gene is usually required so that family members can be offered testing for this mutation. Genetic testing is available mainly from laboratories specializing in porphyria diagnosis. Patients and family members who have inherited porphyria should be counseled on how to limit their risk of future attacks.

The presence of a motor-predominant peripheral neuropathy accompanied by gastrointestinal distress and neuropsychiatric manifestations are strong clues to the diagnosis of porphyria.[8] Recovery of mental function often lags behind physical recovery. Long-term effective management requires avoidance of the factors mentioned previously that can bring upon an attack.

The treatment of AIP is directed toward the specific symptoms that are apparent in each individual. Treatment may require the coordinated efforts of a team of specialists. Pediatricians, neurologists, hematologists, liver specialists, psychiatrists, and other healthcare professionals may need to coordinate an action plan. Genetic counseling may benefit affected individuals and their families.

The objective of treatment is to manage symptoms, prevent complications, and to suppress heme creation (synthesis), which reduces the production of porphyrin precursors. Initial treatment steps also include stopping any medications that can potentially worsen AIP or cause an attack and ensuring proper caloric intake. Individuals who are prone to attacks should eat a normal balanced diet as outlined in chapter 5 and should not restrict their intake of carbohydrates or calories, even for short periods. Patients should avoid smoking, including marijuana, and avoid heavy alcohol intake, as each can induce cytochromes P450. Sources of physical, psychological, and emotional stress should be avoided as much as possible. The many methods of stress reduction mentioned in chapter 7, including meditation, can be helpful. Infection or other illness that can cause metabolic stress can incite an attack; thus, prompt treatment of intercurrent infections or other illnesses with safe antibiotics and hydration is essential. All appropriate vaccinations to prevent infections that may trigger an attack should be administered.

Initial treatment in patients with confirmed acute porphyria without evidence of infection may require hospitalization for fluid hydration and monitoring of vital signs and liver, circulatory, and neurologic function.

Monitoring for and treatment of expected electrolyte abnormalities, including hyponatremia and hypomagnesemia, and seizures are recommended due to possible central nervous system involvement.

Premenstrual attacks often resolve quickly with the onset of menstruation. Some women suffer monthly recurrent attacks during their menstrual cycles and can have symptomatic improvement with birth control medication to suppress ovulation. Others report decreased symptoms when they take low-dose oral contraceptives. Most women with AIP tolerate pregnancy well despite increased serum-circulating progesterone. Some women have more frequent attacks while pregnant; such attacks are treated in the same manner as for non-pregnant women.

Meet Ray

It's not surprising that the diagnosis of porphyria is often missed even when a patient presents to doctors and emergency rooms with potentially life-threatening, recurrent attacks of severe abdominal pain, constipation, tachycardia, and neurological or neuropsychiatric abnormalities. If you believe you are suffering from this disease, you will need to carry a detailed history of porphyrogenic drug exposure so doctors will know how to treat you. The diagnosis and treatment of Lyme disease employing a variety of antibiotics, as with my patient Ray, who had undiagnosed bouts of abdominal pain and progressive nervous system disease, was a tipoff to the diagnosis of AIP.[9]

Ray came to see me complaining of fatigue, abdominal pain, chronic vomiting, urinary retention, weakness, numbness, tingling, lightheadedness, fainting sensation, palpitations, and depression. He was also experiencing progressive weakness, numbness, tingling, and burning sensation of his skin with no apparent physical cause. He also complained of dizziness and heart palpitations. Ray told me that his depression started in high school after a single bout with Lyme disease, for which he was treated with a month of intravenous ceftriaxone. For several years afterward, and while under the care of different Lyme specialists, he received different combinations of antibiotics, antifungals, and antiparasitic treatments. He also experienced frequent abdominal cramping, so severe that he would take himself to the emergency room. When his bladder function deteriorated, the doctors thought he was experiencing recurrent bladder and kidney infections.

On examination in my office, I noticed Ray's weakness in his upper and lower legs, and he told me he felt a vibration accompanied by a cold temperature sensory loss in the legs above the knee. Electromyography and nerve conduction studies showed demyelinating sensorimotor polyneuropathy along the motor nerves of both legs. Autonomic tilt-table tests showed symptomatic orthostatic intolerance. A skin biopsy taken from the calf and thigh showed a loss of small nerve fibers. Muscle showed atrophy of calf muscle fibers. A sample of cerebrospinal fluid obtained by lumbar puncture showed no evidence of infection, but there was an elevated protein level consistent with an autoimmune process. Urinalysis showed increased levels of 5-ALA and PBG, immediately suggesting to me that Ray suffered from AIP.

The first line of treatment was taking Ray off of his current medications and starting again. Once he discontinued the use of the antibiotics, he showed amazing improvement. The antibiotics were the cause of his leg weakness, as his porphyria was interfering with the synthesis and breakdown of his own blood whenever he was taking antibiotics. We were able to change his medications to ones that Ray can tolerate. Not only is his Lyme disease under control, his mood has significantly improved, his strength has improved, and he no longer complains of lightheadedness, fainting sensations, or palpitations.

Chronic Fatigue Syndrome
Relief for Exhausted Patients

Chronic fatigue syndrome (CFS) is a controversial diagnosis because so many people in the medical community do not believe that this syndrome exists. People who have these symptoms are not taken seriously. They don't know why they feel exhausted all the time, but too often, when they go to see a doctor, they will be met with a response like, "it's just stress; it's all in your head." Worse, there is no established nomenclature to describe the multiple types and manifestations of fatigue, and people usually do not feel comfortable making an appointment with a doctor for "just" fatigue. Together, the lack of understanding of the mechanisms of fatigue contributes to poor assessment and treatment strategies, and may make doctors wary of broaching the topic during a typical examination.

CFS was previously known as *myalgic encephalomyelitis* (ME) and is a serious and disabling disorder. It is also known as *systemic exertion intolerance disease* (SEID), emphasizing the central characteristic of the disorder, that exertion of any sort, whether physical, cognitive, or emotional, adversely affects patients in different parts of their body and in diverse aspects of their lives. So-called ME/CFS/SEID affects an estimated 836,000 to 2.5 million individuals in the United States each year, and women are affected more than men with an average age at onset of 33 years. Adolescents are more likely than younger children to have ME/CFS/SEID, yet children as young as 2 years old have developed the illness.[1] A 2011 study in children[2] noted that the disorder accounted for an important cause of unexplained absences from school. What's more, children with ME/CFS/SEID present differently from adults, with more equal gender balance and greater likelihood of sore throat and headaches and an absence of cognitive symptoms, tender lymph nodes, palpitations, dizziness, general malaise, and pain. Reduced ability to function after any kind of activity (physical, cognitive, emotional, or academic pressure)—often referred to as "a crash" by patients—followed by a prolonged recovery is very common. In girls, ME/CFS/SEID symptoms are often worse at or just before their menstrual period.

This disorder was first regarded as a form of muscle fatigability that lasted up to 3 days following minor physical effort before normal muscle function returned. A series of outbreaks first reported at the Royal Free Hospital in London in the mid-twentieth century included patients with malaise, tender lymph nodes, sore throat, pain, and encephalomyelitis.[3] At the same time, two large outbreaks in the United States, characterized by chronic or recurrent debilitating fatigue and various combinations of other symptoms, including sore throat, lymph node pain and tenderness, headache, myalgia, and arthralgia, attracted attention because of its association with Epstein-Barr virus (EBV). Later investigations at the Centers for Disease Control and Prevention (CDC) reached a consensus on the clinical features of the illness, choosing the term CFS, noting that it not only was it more neutral and inclusive, but that Epstein-Barr virus infection did not predate all cases.

The classic diagnosis of ME/CFS/SEID combines all three categories of the nervous system: CNS, PNS, and ANS, in order of symptom prevalence, manifesting neurocognitive deficits, chronic fatigue, and autonomic instability.[4] It is characterized by chronic or recurrent debilitating fatigue and various combinations of other symptoms, including sore throat, lymph node pain and tenderness, headache, myalgia (muscle aches), and arthralgia (joint pain). Sufferers also experience memory and concentration impairments, and confusion. A common symptom of unrefreshing sleep is due to sleep dysfunction or disturbances. Affected children and adults also manifest orthostatic intolerance with disabling cardiovascular, gastrointestinal, and genitourinary impairments.

Dysregulation of the immune system and other metabolic disturbances contribute to this complex syndrome. In many patients, the onset of the disease process can be traced to an infectious trigger such as mononucleosis, stress, an immune deficiency, or autoimmunity.[5] I have also seen a causal link with COVID-19 and the herpes virus and Lyme disease, and the antibodies made to fight it.[6,7,8] ME/CFS/SEID frequently co-occurs with other systemic autoimmune disorders.[9] The term encephalomyelitis refers to an inflammation of the brain and spinal cord, typically due to a viral infection like mononucleosis. Yet the infection could have occurred in the distant past, and patients do not respond to antiviral therapies.

Some people with ME/CFS/SEID have read that their condition may be linked to an immunization. However, testing often shows that these people who coincidentally develop ME/CFS/SEID after immunization typically show evidence of existing altered immunity, not simply against the immunized disorder. Having said that, it is true that post-vaccination adverse immune phenomena can have long latency periods of months to years following immunization, making a cause and effect determination difficult.[10] It is possible that vaccination-induced ME/CFS/SEID may have had indolent or subclinical symptoms that are made more clinically apparent only after immunization due to the immune activation associated with vaccination.

ME/CFS/SEID can begin suddenly, gradually, or with an abrupt increase in the intensity and frequency of milder chronic symptoms. A gradual onset is more common in younger children and can occur over months or years.[11] Mildly affected young people might be able to attend school, but they might have to limit sports, afterschool activities, and have frequent absences. More severely affected young people can become wheelchair dependent and housebound.

Symptoms often fluctuate significantly during the day and from day-to-day. Commonly, patients are slow to get moving upon awakening, with somewhat better function later in the day. The unpredictable level of function from day-to-day can interfere with planning ahead for school attendance, social outings, or family obligations.

THE ROLE OF STRESS
The role of stress in the onset of CFS has been well studied. Investigators[12] have found that patients with ME/CFS/SEID were nine times more likely to experience a traumatic event or difficulty in the 3 months prior to their symptoms, and four times more likely to experience such events 1 year before onset of their illness than a similar population of healthy controls.

The reverse is also true. By mitigating stress you may be able to relieve these symptoms. That does not mean that this disorder is "all in your head." I believe that it is a very real disease process that can be triggered or reinforced by stress.

TESTING FOR ME/CFS/SEID

The pathology of ME/CFS/SEID remains unknown and there is no diagnostic test for the disorder. However, there is a screening system of criteria that you can meet to be diagnosed effectively with this, and to be excluded if you don't have those criteria. Existing diagnostic criteria are purely clinical, which means that a doctor needs to see the symptoms for 6 months before a diagnosis can be made. If you think you might be suffering from ME/CFS/SEID, talk to your doctor about electrodiagnostic studies, including nerve conductions and electromyography, nerve fiber studies, and brain imaging. I also request autonomic tilt-table testing for evidence of hypotension or postural orthostatic tachycardia (POTS) that can contribute to disabling fatigue.

TREATING ME/CFS/SEID

Determining the most effective means of treatment will likely take into account recognition of the natural history of the disease and its temporal progression with or without various empiric treatment regimens, and recognition of subsets of patients with shared disturbances in response to physical and emotional stressors, infection, immune dysfunction, and the expression of associated genetic, epigenetic, and environmental triggers. Successful management is based on determining the optimum balance of rest and activity to help prevent post-exertional symptom worsening. Medications are helpful to treat the symptoms, including pain, insomnia, orthostatic intolerance, and others.

Clinical trials employing the B-cell depleting biological agent rituximab have shown beneficial results in as many as half of severely affected cases. I have also had great success with using intravenous immunoglobulin therapies. This treatment has been well documented over the past 25 years.[13] The efficacy of IVIg supports the concept that immunologic disturbances play an important role in the development of ME/CFS/SEID.

Meet Debbie

Debbie was a 14-year-old, previously healthy girl[14] who developed flu-like symptoms, sore throat, low-grade fever, fatigue, swollen glands, intense headaches, leg weakness, and gait difficulty coincidentally after immunization with the human papilloma virus (HPV). Her mother was sure that the vaccine was the cause of her health issues and came to me to confirm her suspicions. Debbie's mother reported that a month or so following the vaccine her health further worsened, with onset of syncope, a temporary loss of consciousness caused by a fall in blood pressure, and incapacitating chronic fatigue. Debbie was so weak that she began to attend school in a wheelchair. Psychiatric evaluation found no evidence of psychosomatic symptoms, panic, or anxiety disorders. Her bloodwork evaluation revealed an elevated antinuclear antibody titer and weakly possible lupus serology, which meant that she may have an autoimmune connective tissue disorder. She was diagnosed with an undifferentiated connective tissue disease. Serology results for EBV, Lyme, Babesia, and Ehrlichia were all negative. Titers to *Streptococcus pneumonia* indicated previous exposure but were within normal range, thus ruling out recent exposure, but confirming a past infection.

Over the course of her illness, Debbie experienced a complete loss of consciousness approximately 12 times. Autonomic testing showed orthostatic intolerance with prolonged standing, leading to the diagnosis of POTS and ME/CFS/SEID.

Debbie was placed on a POTS protocol, which improved her chronic fatigue, pain, and cognitive function. The mother's concerns about the contribution of the HPV vaccine proved to be valid; however, it was not a simple cause and effect. Instead, HPV inoculation probably contributed to Debbie's genetic background of autoimmune disease, further predisposing her to ME/CFS/SEID.

17

Lyme Disease

The Great Imitator or the Great Trigger?

Lyme disease is a pervasive, epidemic medical problem. It is currently the most commonly reported *tick-borne* disease (TBD) in the United States. Parents, their children, and adults from every walk of life, every part of the country, and around the world have come to see me with a Lyme-related problem. Not only is it so pervasive, it's the perfect example of how I-Cubed can affect brain health.

Lyme disease is a bacterial infection that is transmitted by the bite of Ixodes ticks infected by with the *Borrelia (B.) burgdorferi* spirochete. These hard shell ticks also feed on infected rodents (white-footed mice, squirrels, etc.) and birds in nature, thereby transferring the infection from its source in nature to a human host. Many physicians, including myself, consider Lyme disease to be an important trigger of autoimmunity. The body experiences the infectious reaction to the tick at the same time as it mounts a post-infectious autoimmune response. Factors that contribute to the likelihood of Lyme infectivity also probably related to triggered autoimmunity include age of the patient, the strain of *Borrelia* that the tick carries, the duration of tick attachment, co-infections in the bite, as well as any preexisting immune disorders, and any relevant genetic factors. At the same time, Lyme disease is a master at hiding from the immune system, which is one of the reasons why it is so difficult to treat. This may also be the point where the inflammatory post-infectious autoimmune disease starts and the Lyme infection ends. Even though Lyme has a unique capacity to stay in the body, and has the potential for relapsing and remitting features, I believe its trigger nature activates the immune system, which then launches its own response. Lyme might have been the original insult that activated the immune system, which then caused other neurological issues even after the infection was long gone. This is why I believe that while Lyme disease might be a factor or trigger, it may not be the only cause of autoimmune symptoms and conditions that affect brain health.

However, Lyme disease has been directly connected to changes in brain health. Lyme neuroborreliosis (LNB) is the preferred term for the neuro-inflammatory illness that affects all three systems: CNS, PNS, and ANS as the spirochete following infection. As far back as 2004, researchers were able to prove that spirochetes could travel into the CNS, including the brain and spinal cord, many months after the initial infection. In a more recent 2015 study, the causal role of inflammation in LNB was described in an experimental model of monkeys inoculated with live *B. burgdorferi*. The investigators concluded that infection by *B. burgdorferi* triggers a vigorous post-infectious immune response that leads to the symptoms, signs, and neuropathology that are attributed to the initial infection.

Bannwarth syndrome, a neurological disease characterized as intense nerve pain radiating from the spine, is known to be caused by *B. burgdorferi*, which affects the CNS and PNS at the same time. These sufferers are often mistakenly diagnosed with Guillain-Barre syndrome, a much rarer disorder in which the immune system attacks the nerves.

BE ON THE LOOKOUT FOR THESE LYME DISEASE SYMPTOMS

Lyme disease has long been called the "great imitator," because, like syphilis, it can affect all systems in the brain and the body. It is known to have characteristic dermatologic, rheumatologic, neurologic, and cardiac manifestations. The most common clinical marker for the disease is the bulls-eye, or erythema migrans (EM), rash; this initial skin lesion has been noted in up to three-quarters of confirmed cases. Because Lyme disease can manifest anywhere in the brain or body, symptoms can include:

- Abdominal pain
- Brain fog

- Depression
- Dysesthesia: a painful, itchy, burning, or restrictive sensation caused by nerve damage
- Fatigue
- Fever
- Fibromyalgia: musculoskeletal pain accompanied by fatigue, sleep, memory, and mood issues
- Headache
- Memory difficulty
- Musculoskeletal symptoms: joint swelling, arthritis, painful joints, muscle pain
- Nervous system symptoms: meningitis, encephalitis, cranial neuritis (Bell palsy), radiculoneuritis, and encephalomyelitis
- Palpitations
- Paresthesia: the sensation of tingling, pricking, chilling, burning, or numbness on the skin with no apparent cause
- Peripheral neuropathy
- Sore throat
- Stiff neck

BOX 17.1

LYME DISEASE MISCONCEPTIONS

I see many mothers who strongly believe that they transmitted their own Lyme disease to their child before or during birth. However, this is probably untrue. Most experts agree that Lyme disease is neither contagious nor transmitted in utero or at birth. Lyme disease may look like it clusters in a family, because all members are exposed to the same risk simply by living in the same Lyme-endemic community or by vacationing together.

(Continued)

(*Box 17.1, continued*)

There is also no known prophylactic treatment for Lyme disease. While there still some lingering debate about the effectiveness of a single dose of antibiotic following any given tick bite, you are still better off finding and testing the tick for Lyme disease rather than blindly taking what may very well be an unnecessary course of therapy.

A BRIEF HISTORY OF LYME DISEASE

While the number of Lyme cases overall has not increased, there has been an overall increase in the geographic distribution[3] of the disease. Originally confined to the northeastern United States, by 2013 the ticks carrying Lyme disease could be found in all fifty states, and 95 percent of confirmed cases were reported from 14 northeast and midwestern states including Connecticut, Delaware, Maine, Maryland, Massachusetts, Minnesota, New Hampshire, New Jersey, New York, Pennsylvania, Rhode Island, Vermont, Virginia, and Wisconsin.

Yet while Lyme disease was originally named for Lyme, Connecticut, in 1990s, the disease had been previously found in Europe 50 years earlier. In 1922, the first papers were published in the *Journal de Medicine de Lyon*, France, that reported a meningoradiculitis (meninges and cranial or spinal root) involvement with Lyme disease. The original case[4] describes a 58-year-old man admitted with pain, paralysis, and wasting of the right arm, with left sciatic pain and low back pain. Three months earlier, he had been bitten by a tick on the left buttock, which was the site of later sciatica, followed by radiating pain. An inflammatory ring of skin redness was noted on the left buttock with a bite mark at the ring's center, which later became large, red, and uniform without vesicles and occupying the entire buttock.

In 1944, Bannwarth[5] described 13 patients with non-infectious meningitis accompanied by root pain and sensory and motor loss, and palsy of the facial nerve. Sköldenberg and colleagues[6] characterized EM and the bull's eye rash that occurs in the summer or fall due to a preceding tick bite. Such patients develop later fatigue, malaise, weight loss, and fever, followed by facial nerve paralysis and motor and peripheral neuropathy. Noting antibodies against *Ixodes dammini* spirochetes in the cerebrospinal fluid (CSF) of three patients, and a favorable response to a 2-week course of intravenous penicillin, these researchers further[4] postulated that the cause was a European bacteria, delivered via a vector.

In 1972, Lyme arthritis became a newly formed term to describe inflammatory arthritis found in Lyme, Connecticut. Researchers found that the incidences of the disease grew in the summer and early fall.[7,8] In 1977, Steere and colleagues[10] studied three closely situated Connecticut communities with a geographic clustering of Lyme disease cases that suggested an insect vector again had transmitted the infection to humans.

Two years later, Reik and colleagues[9] summarized the neurological abnormalities of Lyme disease in a cohort of cases diagnosed by the presence of EM and arthritis, half of whom recall being bitten by ticks, up to 20 days before onset of symptoms. In 1982, Burgdorfer and colleagues[5] isolated the *Borrelia* bacteria carried by *Ixodes dammini* ticks. They noted that Lyme-specific immunoglobulin (Ig)M antibody titers reached a peak between the third and sixth week after onset of the disease, whereas specific IgG antibody titers rise more slowly, becoming highest only months later when arthritis symptoms presented. The practice of obtaining antibody titers during what was thought of at the time as the recovery period allowed researchers to see how the immune system transforms from a rapid and early IgM response to a long-lasting IgG response, which is how the immune system is supposed to do its job. It also tells us how early the immune system kicks in, and therefore how soon autoimmunity could potentially lead to its own symptoms through the process of I-Cubed. The expected IgM to IgG transformation assures the clinician that the patient has a true positive IgM result as it migrates to IgG because, and in the absence thereof, testing might be interpreted as a false positive for the disease.

A few years later, Pachner and Steere[10] were the first to study patients with neurological manifestations of Lyme disease. In 34 of the 38 patients, they found that the first stage of the illness included symptoms of malaise, fatigue, headache, stiff neck, fever, myalgia, arthralgia, dysesthesia, sore throat, and abdominal pain. A second stage of neurological manifestations commences a month later with a characteristic triad of meningitis, cranial neuritis, and radiculoneuritis. In 1987, Halperin and colleagues[11] summarized the PNS manifestations; their observations led them to conclude that many patients with Lyme disease have significant PNS abnormalities that may resolve with prompt early antibiotic treatment, yet may still experience later PNS involvement that improves only after both antibiotics and immune-modulatory therapy are included in the plan to treat immune-mediated damage to the nerves.

In 1989, the same investigators[12] determined that in rare cases, symptoms of a multiple sclerosis (MS)-like illness and psychiatric disorders appeared. The patients with encephalopathy or focal CNS disease have evidence of intrathecal synthesis of B. burgdorferi–specific antibodies. The authors concluded that a Lyme infection could be a cause of encephalopathy.

In 1989, Steere[13] summarized the causation, vector and animal hosts, clinical manifestations, pathogenesis, and treatment of human Lyme disease. He noted that there were in fact three stages of infection, each with different clinical manifestations, and his model is what we now use to individualize a treatment protocol for every patient with Lyme:

- *Stage 1* follows the tick bite with the spread of B. burgdorferi bacteria locally in the skin, producing in 60 percent to 80 percent of patients an EM rash that fades in 3 to 4 weeks, and could be accompanied by fever, minor constitutional symptoms, or regional adenopathy (swollen glands and/or lymph nodes).
- *Stage 2* occurs in the following days or weeks after the tick bite, when the bacteria has spread via the bloodstream to distant organ sites including the brain, myocardium, retina, muscle, bone, synovium (the soft tissue that lines the joints), spleen, and liver, where symptoms can start to emerge.
- Late infection characterizes *Stage 3* disease that includes episodes of arthritis lasting months rather than weeks, and can become chronic. Lymphocytic meningitis occurs several weeks after the skin rash and is characterized by varying degrees of headache, neck stiffness, and photophobia (a discomfort or pain to the eyes due to light exposure). Other symptoms emerge including progressive encephalomyelitis,[14] subacute encephalitis, dementia, and demyelinating diseases.[15] In 1990, Logigian and colleagues[16] defined chronic Lyme disease as a disorder where Lyme symptoms continue to occur 12 months after Stage 1. However, that term has been replaced by post-treatment Lyme disease syndrome (PTLDS) and reserved for those

who continue to test positive using screening tests, even after a standard of care course of antibiotics, reflecting the presence of non-viable spirochetes or their remnants.

DIAGNOSING LYME DISEASE IS DIFFICULT

Lyme disease is difficult to detect because the spirochete is a master at hiding from the immune system, making routine testing inexact. What's more, without evidence of a bull's eye or EM rash, joint pain, meningitis, or facial palsy, Lyme is actually very hard to catch. The tests for Lyme disease generally do not go beyond registering exposure to the organism or the immune response: they can only prove that at some point, you had been exposed to the organism, and you engaged an immune response. These tests do not show if the disease is still active.

According to the CDC, Lyme disease should only be diagnosed with a positive *B. burgdorferi* culture, two-tier test, or isolated IgG or IgM Western blot seropositivity. An active case of LNB can only be confirmed if the CSF shows positivity for *B. burgdorferi* antibodies in greater levels than what can be found in the bloodstream reflected in a positive Lyme Index (LI) >1.1, which is the most predictive index for Lyme disease. It goes beyond the serum titers; it goes beyond seeing a Western blot in the spinal fluid.

Brain and spinal cord MRI can determine if there are white matter changes and gray matter atrophy. Conventional MRI can show subcortical white matter lesions, while high-field three-dimensional proton MRI spectroscopy can assess key brain metabolites including N-acetylaspartate (NAA) levels, an indicator of neuronal integrity.[17]

Nuclear medicine brain SPECT imaging can reveal various patterns of blood flow in various stages of encephalopathy due to infectious or inflammatory disruption of the BBB.[18] Brain PET imaging is useful in the evaluation of cognitive and memory disturbances. Experimentally, PET has been used to assess post-infectious (I-Cubed) cortical brain immunity in patients with PTLDS. Brain PET/MRI may be used to precisely locate areas of hypometabolism that correlate with cognitive and neuropsychiatric deficits.

I have also found that in the most severe cases involving the CNS, a lumbar puncture to obtain CSF offers the best way of identifying LNB with certainty.[19] Common CSF findings include elevated protein content, normal glucose, lymphocytic pleocytosis, and humoral immune response composed

---

BOX 17.2

BEWARE OF COINFECTIONS

According to Lyme disease expert Dr. Richard Horowitz, author of *Why Can't I Get Better?* and *How Can I Get Better?*,[21] there are hundreds of species of *Borrelia*, so when we talk about "Lyme disease" we are really talking about a disease complex caused by a large family of bacteria. For example, if you see an EM rash on your body, it could have been caused by more than one species of *Borrelia*. What's more, the same ticks carrying *Borrelia* may also be carrying other infections, including *Bartonella*, which cause stretch marks on different parts of the body. Other tick-borne infections like *Ehrlichiosis* can cause either a flat or raised rash, while Rocky Mountain spotted fever can cause small red spots to appear.[22]

---

of *Borrelia*-specific antibodies that depend upon the stage and activity of the disorder.[20] Detecting any or all of these abnormalities in the CSF makes the case for potentially active LNB that necessitates intravenous antibiotics and immune modulatory (Ig) therapy, in that order.

TREATING LYME DISEASE

The most effective antibiotics for treating Lyme disease include doxycycline, amoxicillin, cefuroxime, and ceftriaxone, respectively, for localized early or late-stage systemic and nervous system manifestations. The three neurological syndromes clearly attributed to Lyme disease include lymphocytic meningitis, painful radiculoneuritis, and encephalomyelitis, each of which require immediate antibiotic treatment to forestall clinical worsening.

The overall TAPES approach means looking at different areas of your life to find sources of unnecessary inflammation and neurotoxicity that may impair your immunity and slow your recovery from infections like Lyme disease. When dealing with Lyme, look at every aspect of this protocol. Are you following an anti-inflammatory diet and removing known food allergies or sensitivities, including gluten, dairy, and refined sugar? Can you reintroduce some type of exercise that will not cause pain? Can you try relieving stress through meditation or other types of cognitive behavioral therapies? Have you evaluated the possibility of mold in your home?

Treatment regimens for the neurological manifestations of Lyme disease are summarized in the following. The categories (first line, second line, etc.) refer to my first choice of medications (and then second choice, etc.) based on empiric efficacy according to Clinical Guidelines of the American Academy of Neurology (AAN) for the Treatment of Nervous System Lyme Disease:[23]

Suggested Treatment Based on Neurological Syndrome[24]

Meningitis: IV ceftriaxone, cefotaxime, or penicillin G
Encephalomyelitis: IV ceftriaxone, cefotaxime, or penicillin G
Encephalopathy: treat as encephalomyelitis if CSF abnormal; IV or orally antibiotics if CSF normal
PNS radiculopathy, neuropathy, mononeuritis multiplex, cranial neuritis: oral antibiotics or IV if treatment failure

Suggested Treatment Regimens

First Line

Oral adult regimen: doxycycline 100–200 mg BID
Intravenous adult regimen: ceftriaxone 2 grams IV daily
Oral pediatric regimen (in children years of age or older): doxycycline 4–8 mg/kg/d in divided doses max 200 mg/dose
Intravenous pediatric regimen: ceftriaxone 50–75 mg/kg/d in one dose; max 2 grams

Second Line

Oral adult regimen (when doxycycline contraindicated): amoxicillin 500 mg TID
Intravenous adult regimen: cefotaxime 2 grams IV Q8H
Oral pediatric regimen (when doxycycline contraindicated): amoxicillin 50 mg/kg/d in three divided doses; max 500 mg/dose
Intravenous pediatric regimen: cefotaxime 150–200 mg/kg/d in three or four divided doses; max 6 grams/day

Third Line

Oral adult regimen (when doxycycline contraindicated): cefuroxime axetil 500 mg BID
Intravenous adult regimen: penicillin G 18–24 MU/day, divided doses Q4H

Oral pediatric regimen (when doxycycline contraindicated): cefuroxime axetil
30 mg/kg/d in two divided doses; max 500 mg/dose
Intravenous pediatric regimen: penicillin G 200–400 MU/kg/d in divided doses
Q4H; max 18–24 MU/day

Meet Lucy

Lucy, a 31-year-old financial analyst and exercise enthusiast, suffered from recurring postpartum depression following the births of each of her children. Yet one evening several months following her last pregnancy, she woke up in the middle of the night with pain in her arms. She told me that at first the pain was stronger than a typical gym injury: it seemed to attack all of her joints with an intensity that electrified her body. The only thing that relieved the pain was running cold water over her hands.

Over the next few weeks she saw a multitude of doctors specializing in neurology, rheumatology, infectious disease, pain management, and physical therapy, but the best they could do was prescribe oxycodone and morphine, commenting that whatever the cause, it was probably not in their specialty. She soon became addicted to these opioid medications, yet the pain was so intense she was not able to go back to work. Her husband had to take a family medical leave from work to care of her and the kids.

When the pain migrated to her legs, Lucy was advised to have a blood test for Lyme disease. She checked into the hospital where she underwent a comprehensive evaluation without a clear path forward. While in the hospital, her husband called me, asking for a meeting. He explained her symptoms and after speaking with her medical team, we decided that she was stable enough to leave the hospital and come directly to my office.

Lucy was extremely anxious and unable to keep her hands calm during our first office visit. I performed an electromyography and nerve conductions, left calf and thigh skin biopsies for epidermal nerve fiber densities, a tilt-table test, and ordered additional blood tests when it became evident that her symptoms were due to Lyme exposure, resulting in painful POTS, OCD, and depression, a trifecta of the CNS, PNS, and ANS involvement triggered by untreated Lyme disease for a year or more.

Lucy started taking doxycycline and IVIg therapy, and I advised her to obtain certification for medical cannabis because I was very concerned about the long-term consequences of opioids. I suggested that she see a psychiatrist who agreed to supervise her opioid detoxification and to prescribe an antidepressant as well as insight-oriented psychotherapy. Two weeks free of opioids and taking the right medications, Lucy was 85 percent back to normal.

Spondyloarthropathy

I-Cubed and Genetically Predetermined Joint Diseases

Both patients and physicians have a difficult time understanding how joint pain, often referred to as arthralgia, can be at the same time post-infectious, inflammatory, and autoimmune as well as genetically predetermined. The answer is the inconspicuous role infection, the immune system, and genetics play in triggering a group of joint disorders referred to as spondyloarthropathy (SpA) that includes reactive arthritis (ReA) and ankylosing spondylitis.[1] Yet the story becomes even more interesting when you consider that fatigue due to altered CNS function significantly adds to the disability of SpAs and may be an early clue to its diagnosis. In fact, arthralgia and fatigue due to brain dysfunction improve significantly with immune modulatory therapy and a TAPES lifestyle.

UNDERSTANDING JOINT PAIN

Pain-sensitive tissues are the source of joint pain, and when they are severely affected can lead to disability, psychological distress, and impaired quality of life. These pain-sensitive structures, all innervated by nerve elements, reside in ligaments, tendons, bone, and connective tissue comprising the intra-articular or inner portion of the joint, and the extra-articular or outcome areas surrounding the joint. Inflammatory mediators inside the joint that sensitize pain receptors enhance the feeling of pain transmitted from a joint along peripheral and CNS pathways.[2] A more centralized pain results both from the lowering of thresholds and inhibition in the CNS to more prolonged and intense pain,[3] and for that reason pain may not always be easily pinpointed to a given joint.

Pain in SpA is usually attributed to inflammation. However, treatment with potent biologic agents that control inflammation does not always control the pain. Pain is hence likely to be multifactorial. Fatigue is another prominent feature of this condition, which again tends to respond poorly to potent biologic agents. Advances in neuroimaging have helped in better understanding the dynamic nature of brain networks in the perception of pain. Animal models have helped in developing concepts of peripheral and central sensitization in pain transmission.[4]

Pain management includes a combination of physical therapy for muscle and soft tissues, drugs such as muscle relaxants and centrally acting analgesics, and cognitive behavioral therapy.[5] Controlling pain within the joint requires injections, systemic analgesics and anti-inflammatory medication, and arthroscopic repair or joint replacement when irreparable damage has occurred. Yet even before contemplating the mode of pain management, an important question is whether the joint disorder falls into the category of a SpA, requiring more precise diagnosis and treatment.

When overlapping vertebral joints are the site of focal or widespread inflammation, back pain develops. However, the pain of SpA differs from mechanical back pain. SpA is diagnosed by its insidious onset, history of morning stiffness, pain at night, and association with a recent infection. While typically self-limited, resolving in weeks to months, a proportion of individuals with ReA develop persistent symptoms. Symptoms include asymmetric large joint pain and extra-articular features including tendinitis, eye involvement (uveitis), and a variety of skin rashes. Both mechanical back pain and SpA disorders improve with exercise and show a favorable response to nonsteroidal anti-inflammatory drugs (NSAIDs).

The fatigue in SpA, like central pain, has a CNS neural basis. Patients with SpA usually have neuropathic pain, with loss of joint position sensation, and decreased mechanical and thermal sensitivity in the joint and overlying skin.[6] Both pain and sensory loss cause fatigue and deficits in attention[7] due to CNS mechanisms by affecting areas of the brain associated with executive functioning. Subjects with inflammatory joint pain have significant fatigue that correlates with disease activity and measures of their emotional strength and spinal mobility. Moreover, a higher score of fatigue in such patients correlates positively with well-developed executive control networks of the brain as shown on MRI that suggests the importance of attentional and memory mechanisms of sensory experiences, including pain, respectively located in the frontal lobe and hippocampus.

Some types of SpAs show a strong causal relationship with infections. Septic arthritis, for instance, directly results from joint infection by pathogenic microorganisms, whereas the synovial fluid cultures in ReA are sterile, implying the likelihood of a predominant autoimmune pathogenesis.

So where do these illnesses begin? One mechanism is the persistence of microbial agents due to an unresolved active infection somewhere in the body; when detected by the immune system, this triggers an exaggerated immune response.

A second cause is the intracellular uptake and trafficking of bacteria within the joint synovium that leads to inflammation. This differs from the first cause in that the microbes make their way into the joint space or fluid, inciting local damage and an immune response.

A third explanation is the process of molecular mimicry, whereby bacterial agents cause an immune response that targets normal body antigens that resemble the infectious intruder, which in this case is the affected joint.

A fourth mechanism is the activity of autoimmunity associated with specialized receptors located on T-cells, called Toll receptors, that recognize bacterial ligands and activate a separate potent immune cell response.

THE GUT–BRAIN CONNECTION INFLUENCES YOUR JOINTS

A fifth suggestion is the role that gastrointestinal infection can play. Studies have found that infections that lead to increased intestinal permeability allow certain antigens to interact with the immune system and cause joint inflammation,[8] particularly in the synovial fluid.[9] One study found that the synovial fluid of individuals with ReA contained bacterial DNA, antigenic proteins, and lipopolysaccharides. What's more, the host genetics, independent of HLA-B27, contributes to the population of microorganisms that reside in the gut.

In animal experiments, mice that are genetically prone to colitis or inflammation of the intestines, later develop SpA when colonized with *Bacterioides* organisms. This story became even more interesting when the same animals exhibited signs of activated T-helper cell immunity and the HLA-B27 genotype, with a further heightening of the immune response to interleukin (IL)-23-protein production. Taken together, these findings suggest that genetically pre-disposed animals react to microbial imbalance by altering their immune system in the intestines and creating an inflammatory state. The process is mediated by T-cell and IL production, which ultimately leads to local and systemic clinical disease manifested as a SpA-like illness.

SIGNIFICANCE OF GENETIC PREDETERMINATION BY HLA-B27

SpA diseases have a strong genetic component. Many of those affected typically carry the HLA-B27 gene, whose presence is a tip-off for the risk for joint inflammation and a host of associated neuroinflammatory manifestations. For instance, HLA-B27 is associated with a range of neurological problems including cognitive issues, neuropathy, and dysautonomia.[10]

Genetic testing for HLA-B27 is key for diagnosing patients with ankylosing spondylitis, which occurs when there is the presence of over two dozen genes that together with HLA-B27 result in a chronic inflammatory disease that affects the joints.[11] The population prevalence of HLA-B27 and particular types of SpA, like ReA, vary depending upon whether the gene is present or expressed in given individuals. HLA-B27 is highly prevalent in Caucasian Northern Europeans, even though it is virtually absent in other populations that develop ReA. In fact, several epidemiologic studies estimate that no more than half of individuals who develop ReA are HLA-B27 positive.[12]

Experimental mice with the HLA-B27 genotype[13] that later develop colitis and SpA when colonized with certain bacterial flora increase the colonic expression of cytokines compared with experimentally germ-free animals.[14] Such animals show activation of helper T-cells[15] with alterations (misfolding) in the HLA-B27 gene that further heightens the immune response associated with increased IL-23 production.[16] Taken together, these findings suggest that genetically predisposed animals react to a microbial imbalance by altering their immune system in the intestinal compartment toward a more inflammatory state. The process is mediated by T-cell and IL production, which ultimately leads to local and systemic clinical disease manifested as a SpA-like human illness.[17]

TREATING SPA

Besides genetic testing, neuroimaging is an important tool for establishing a diagnosis of SpA. Conventional x-rays, ultrasound, MRI, SPECT, and skeletal bone scan studies can all detect joint damage and inflammation. These tests are also useful for predicting outcomes and response to treatments. Once identified, the optimal management of patients with SpA requires a combination of pharmacological and non-pharmacological approaches. To emphasize this point, best practice guidelines from the National Ankylosing Spondylitis Society recommend that patients should have access to a multidisciplinary team offering a full range of appropriate services in a timely manner.[18] The aim of all interventions should be to maximize quality of life and functional capacity.

Continuous treatment of patients with persistently active, symptomatic disease with appropriate and safe doses of NSAIDs is the recommended first-line treatment for all symptomatic patients unless contraindicated. Substantial relief of symptoms, including back pain and stiffness, is seen in up to 80 percent of patients receiving NSAIDs.[19] These treatments also enhance physiotherapy because maximal reductions in pain and stiffness are required to achieve the optimal benefit from physiotherapy. However, only one-third of patients achieve partial remission with NSAIDs alone.[20] Synthetic and biologic disease modifying drug therapy is advocated in severe cases. Adalimumab, a fully human recombinant IgG1 monoclonal antibody that specifically targets the cytokine tumor necrosis factor, was associated with sustained reduction in symptoms and signs of SpA in 58 percent of patients. Empiric broad-spectrum antibiotics do not appear to have a therapeutic role. However, bacterial modulation through fecal microbial transplantation to restore a healthier intestinal microbiome are showing promising results. Its role in SpA is unclear and should probably only be considered when there is concomitant irritable bowel disease or other types of colitis.

Regular physical exercise is the cornerstone of optimal treatment for SpA, as it promotes improved muscle strength, joint flexibility, and motor performance, which together may lessen chronic joint pain and discomfort.[21] In the acute phase of joint injury that often accompanies SpA, a program of medically monitored physical therapy is essential to return the joint to a more normal function unit and to offset further damage. Physical therapy can also address balance issues that accompany SpA.

In addition, joining a support group is a great idea. Being with others who have the same symptoms and experiences has the potential to improve motivation and compliance within the context of a long-term condition.

WHEN HYPERMOBILITY OCCURS WITH JOINT STIFFNESS

SpA is normally thought to be associated with joint stiffness or total body stiffness. Typically, the usual findings include having a "bamboo rod" looking spine on standard x-ray. These people walk in a stiff and imbalanced manner. Yet there are cases where joint stiffness is overshadowed by joint laxity or hypermobility.[22] Although rare, it shows how difficult diagnosis and management may be. People with hypermobility, like those who suffer from POTS, are more likely to be injured or suffer repeated injuries and dislocations. This may be why this subgroup of patients that exhibit both SpA and joint hypermobility are more prone to anxiety, depression, and fatigue, which may exacerbate their symptoms.

A patient, Bobby, had lax, stretchy skin since birth and later developed shoulder, femoral, and knee hyperextensibility and instability. Arthralgia symptoms were evident during adolescence and progressed to inflammatory back pain with morning stiffness, as well as fatigue and anxiety that exacerbated in adulthood. He was HLA-B27 positive. Treatment with NSAIDs and the anti-inflammatory sulfasalazine (Azulfidine) resulted in a significant decrease in back pain, and his fatigue and anxiety went away.

Joint hypermobility associated with Ehlers-Danlos syndrome (EDS) is caused by mutations in genes coding for collagen proteins associated with collagen processing and the production of extracellular matrix components. There are six types of this disease, and all involve tissue fragility. The hypermobility type of EDS (HEDS, also known as EDS Type III) is largely characterized by extreme joint laxity and soft, velvety skin. Joint hypermobility is most pronounced in childhood, and individuals with joint hypermobility are colloquially known as being "double jointed." Afflicted individuals are often treated as a curiosity and may even find their increased flexibility a boon in athletic endeavors.

Due to joint instability, HEDS patients suffer from frequent joint stress and injury, leading to chronic arthralgia, soft-tissue rheumatism (i.e., tendonitis, bursitis, epicondylitis), and myalgia; many also suffer from frequent dislocations. Such patients are often afflicted with a plethora of non-musculoskeletal symptoms, such as dysautonomia (POTS), abnormal proprioception, headaches, and gastrointestinal dysmotility, which may lead to nutritional deficits. Many of those with HEDS also suffer from mood disorders, including depression and anxiety.

Scientists now recognize that HEDS is associated with a number of rheumatological conditions, both inflammatory and non-inflammatory, including SpA.[23]

19

Autoimmune Encephalitis

A Brain on Fire

The role autoimmunity plays in neuropsychiatric illnesses has been investigated for decades, ever since the 1930s when autoantibodies were first found in a schizophrenia patient.[1] Since that time, there have been reports of specific autoimmune responses that lead to psychosis, bipolar disease, severe depression, and other neurobehavioral abnormalities.[2] These responses are now referred to as autoimmune encephalitis (AE), a disorder that was first brought to the public's attention by *New York Post* writer Susannah Cahalan's struggle.

Considered a rare diagnosis in 2012, her book, *Brain on Fire*,[3] shows how the manifestations of this disease, which occurred within just 1 month, were caused by a newly described circulating antineuronal antibody to the N-methyl-D-aspartate (NMDA) receptor found in the brain. In 2009, Susannah was a healthy 24-year-old reporter when she began to experience numbness, paranoia, sensitivity to light, and erratic behavior. She first wrote off her symptoms to stress, until she began to experience seizures, hallucinations, and increasingly psychotic behavior. In the hospital, tests revealed that she had high titers of NMDA receptor antibodies in the bloodstream that were targeting neurons after crossing the BBB, leading to her brain illness. However, the process of the damage was reversible with immune-modulatory therapy to counteract the autoimmune attack.

The clinical picture of a patient with anti-NMDA receptor AE looks like someone with a psychiatric disorder.[4] Most patients, like Susannah, appear confused, restless, agitated, with frequent paranoid or delusional thoughts, and alternating episodes of quiet staring and catatonic postures. Testing of the cerebrospinal fluid (CSF) typically shows inflammatory abnormalities, and brain MRI may be normal or show cortical or cerebellar abnormalities, or temporal lobe lesions. One-half of cases are associated with a tumor, typically of the ovary, sometimes masquerading as an ovarian cyst. Although potentially lethal, if sufferers are properly diagnosed and treated, this catastrophic disorder is reversible, as in Susannah Cahalan's story.

Meet Alexandra

Alexandra, a 34-year-old woman, was complaining of headache, feeling feverish, and an overall feeling of being unsure of herself, which was not in her typical nature. She attributed these symptoms to stress and anxiety, and when they didn't resolve within a week, she went ahead and took her husband's anti-anxiety medication one afternoon. The following day her symptoms worsened to the point where she needed to go to the emergency room, where she had convulsions. A brain CT was unremarkable, yet her CSF showed inflammation. MRI of the brain showed bilateral medial temporal lobe lesions notably involving the left hippocampus. An electroencephalogram (EEG) showed mild slowing. Her mental status improved, and she went home with a prescription for anticonvulsants. Yet the next evening Alex woke up in the middle of the night with delusional thoughts.

Over the next few days, she became catatonic and her husband brought her back to the hospital, where she was placed in the intensive care unit. An EEG was ordered to detect the cause of her seizures. A CT and pelvic ultrasound revealed a calcified calcified tumor of her left ovary, a teratoma. Antibodies to NMDA receptor were found in the blood and CSF.

Given the rapid deterioration of her condition, Alex's doctor suggested that her left ovary be removed. She was given intravenous methylprednisolone and plasma exchange followed by IVIg therapy for the next 5 days. One week later, the abnormal movements subsided and the cardiac arrhythmia resolved. She gradually became more alert, yet had no memory of the preceding 2 months. By 2 months after discharge, follow-up MRI revealed considerable improvement in the hippocampus, and her cognitive functions, memory, and psychiatric evaluation were normal. A close examination of the tumor pathology revealed that it expressed NMDA receptors identical to neurons,[5] making this a "paraneoplastic" or cancer-related syndrome. It turns out only a small percentage of cases of NMDA receptor autoantibody-associated AE are paraneoplastic, but their occurrence nonetheless mandates a screen for cancer.

OTHER AUTOANTIBODIES LINKED TO AE

Researchers[6] have described the pathologic features of AE, establishing two main categories of autoantibodies, depending upon whether it targets neuronal antigens located on the surface of neurons (SAg, or Type I) or intracellularly (IAg, or Type II). Two other categories can be postulated: Type III, associated with NMDA receptor antibodies where the antigen is found initially on the surface and later migrates inside the cell; and Type IV, when there is clinically apparent AE without a known autoantibody.

Type I

AE Type I occurs when the putative circulating autoantibody in the blood, targets an antigen on the surface of the brain's neurons, or the brain scaffolding systems, such as the one associated with the voltage-gated potassium channel-complex (VGKC). Brain scaffolding theory[7] suggests that these are molecules that sustain the neural circuits which are important in synapse formation and neural plasticity. When these neurons are attacked by the VGKC antibody, the autoantibody-mediated neuro-inflammatory response begins, disrupting this protective scaffold. Bennett and Vincent[8] conjecture that VGKC-complex antibodies themselves increase the excitability of the brain.

Not so different from the neurological disorder due to increased antibodies to NMDA receptors, patients with VGKC antibodies also present with irritability, depression, hallucinations, personality disturbances, short-term memory loss, sleep disturbances, seizures, variable neuropathy, and dysautonomia. Lahoria and coworkers[9] described Type I AE patients with painful neuropathy. Autonomic involvement is noted in a third of reported cases[10] and is associated with small fiber neuropathy. Immunotherapy employing corticosteroids, IVIg, plasma exchange, or the B-cell depleting immunosuppressant Rituxan has been associated with favorable responses in reducing attacks.

There is recent interest in understanding the neurobiological significance of the VGKC antibody in other seizure disorders, including autosomal dominant lateral temporal epilepsy. Like AE, this disorder is characterized by partial seizures and preceding auditory signs. However, unlike AE, there is a related genetic mutation for this disorder, which is found on chromosome 10q24. This mutation is the underlying molecular mechanism that causes abnormal hippocampal excitability and seizures.[11]

Meet Camille

I had the opportunity to treat Camille, a 68-year-old woman who complained of chronic lightheadedness and palpitations as well as neuropathic pain, numbness, tingling, and weakness of the limbs. She became more concerned when her symptoms worsened to include unprovoked seizure-like episodes of vocalizations, facial grimacing, involuntary head turning, neck stiffness, and left arm posturing lasting a few seconds, which occurred up to a dozen times per day. She also noted progressive memory loss and personality change.

I ordered an EEG to look for the source of her convulsions, but it returned normal. Electromyography and nerve conduction studies showed a peripheral demyelinating neuropathy in her legs. Her skin biopsies showed reduced numbers of epidermal nerve fibers. These findings together indicated autoimmune small fiber neuropathy and large fiber demyelinating polyneuropathy.

Autonomic studies with tilt-table testing showed an immediate fall of her systolic blood pressure, leading me to diagnose autoimmune dysautonomia. Although brain MRI was normal, PET and SPECT showed hypoperfusion in the left frontal and parietal lobes consistent with disruption of the BBB.

Her cerebrospinal fluid was normal. Blood forwarded to the Mayo Clinic in August 2016 showed an elevated titer of VGKC-complex antibody. I witnessed a brief attack where Camille began vocal grunting, facial grimacing, left head turning, neck stiffness, and left arm posturing lasting a few seconds without shaking movements of the limbs, loss of consciousness, or amnesia for the event. The scientific literature refers to them as faciobrachial dystonic seizures.

We started her on a high dose IVIg, and she showed improvement within a few months. Today, she no longer has seizures and her neuropsychiatric complaints have all but disappeared, including her symptoms of neuropathy and dysautonomia.[12]

AE Type II: GAD65-Associated AE Targets an Intraneuronal Antigen

Another type of AE occurs with the GAD65-antibody that attacks an antigen found inside neurons, instead of on their surface. Studies have noted greater numbers of T-cells inflaming neurons in the hippocampus (and related limbic connections) and neuronal cell loss in IAg (AE Type I) compared to the SAg (Type II) cases. Type II AE is more severe than Type I. The most common presenting clinical feature of Type II AE are seizures, followed by cognitive impairment affecting memory, language, executive function, and attention.

Other psychiatric symptoms occur in a third of cases, including depression, behavior, perception, and anxiety. Other less common clinical manifestations are fever, dysautonomia, cerebellar incoordination, and headache. The dominant symptom of seizures and neurocognitive/neuropsychiatric disturbances in most patients with GAD65-autoantibody AE is explained by the frequent involvement of the medial temporal lobes. Brain MRI can confirm abnormalities in the medial temporal lobes, and EEG can reveal temporal lobe epileptic or slow-wave activity. Increased levels of GAD65 autoantibodies are present in the bloodstream. Most patients will not have an underlying malignancy.

Full recovery occurs in about 10 percent with corticosteroids alone, with IVIg, or in combination with plasma exchange. Unrecognized and therefore untreated, the disease can be fatal.

Type IV Seronegative AE

AE can be easy to identify when the autoantibodies appear in testing. However, there is a last type of AE that antibody panels cannot pick up. This type is referred to as seronegative AE, because there is no detectable antibody, yet the same telltale symptoms include cognitive and neuropsychiatric symptoms in addition to seizures that occur in the medial temporal lobe. In these instances, the cause can be traced to circulating antibodies, as in cases of Hashimoto's encephalopathy, or Celiac disease associated with the autoimmune response to gluten, and each with varying potential to direct an autoimmune attack on the brain, culminating in AE.

Because bloodwork is inconclusive, physicians must instead rely on brain PET/MRI to show the metabolic temporal lobe abnormalities. EEG may be useful in classifying the seizure type and establishing the possible need for anticonvulsants with someone with subclinical or inapparent seizures (no disturbance of consciousness or convulsions). IVIg therapy treats this type of AE.

Meet Carl

My patient Carl was 14 years old when he was diagnosed with seronegative AE. He had life-long hypotonia, an abnormally low level of muscle tone, and severe colic as an infant. There was a family history of Celiac disease, and he was suspected of the same. At age 8, he was found to have a bull's eye rash on his belly, and he was treated with doxycycline for 3 months and later herbals and gluten-free diet for optimal health. At age 10, he fell on the gym floor striking his head. At age 12, he developed pain in the right ankle, followed later by weakness of the foot and tremor of the hands.

At the same time Carl began having cognitive and neurobehavioral issues, including depression, agitation, and palpitations. At that time, his cognitive symptoms were connected to Lyme disease, and he was treated with 18 months of the Cowden protocol. During that time he fainted again at school, striking his head on a metal bench. He was also diagnosed with POTS and Hashimoto's thyroiditis.

I performed an electromyography and nerve conduction study of the legs that showed moderately severe distal acquired demyelinating neuropathy. Autonomic studies showed orthostatic tachycardia that compensated for a bout of hypotension when he was tilted head up, not POTS strictly speaking. He was positive for the Celiac DQ2 genotype. PET/MRI of the brain showed a multitude of abnormalities including hypometabolism and structural changes, with signs of early sclerosis due to AE-mediated inflammation. This pointed to the fact that Carl's case was severe despite his young age. EEG monitoring supported the diagnosis of AE, as it revealed a seizure focus.

Carl's case of AE was probably more severe because of the combination of Celiac disease, childhood-onset Lyme disease, and two concussive head injuries leading to cognitive, neuropsychiatric disturbances, brain hypometabolism, and seizure focus, emblematic of AE without a definable autoantibody. He was placed on IVIg and plans to start rituximab to affect a full cure and forestall further deterioration.

Alzheimer's Disease and Other Dementias

Autoimmune Insights

The symptoms of Alzheimer's disease (AD) do not look like the forgetfulness of misplacing your keys. It's when you lose the ability to turn a key or can't remember the multiple steps it takes to complete a task. It is the prototypical dementing disorder and is a neurodegenerative illness that is genetic in nature. AD develops when extracellular amyloid beta (Aβ) plaques and tau proteins accumulate in the brain and form intracellular neurofibrillary tangles.[1] We don't exactly know what the consequences of these plaques or tangle are in terms of altering memory, if it's a toxic effect, or if it's just taking the space of normal brain. However, we do know that as these plaques and tangles increase in volume, AD symptoms become more severe. Interestingly, tau protein buildup has also recently been found in patients with traumatic brain injury (TBI) and concussion.

An investigation of AD brain lesions shows that there may be many sources of immune stimulation that can worsen the condition or produce further deterioration. For example, diabetes, which is autoimmune by nature, and insulin deficiency are connected to a buildup of Aβ protein in the bloodstream, cerebrospinal fluid (CSF), and brain. Antidiabetic therapies in patients with diabetes and cognitive impairment have been shown to be beneficial. I believe this to be related to the anti-inflammatory properties of these drugs, which are immune-modulatory therapies.

Investigators have long suspected that pathogenic microbes might contribute to the onset and progression of AD. Recently, researchers[2] have found that cases of late-onset AD studied at autopsy showed human herpes virus (HHV) 6A and 7 in at least four brain regions. Patients who have Creutzfeldt Jakob disease, a prion illness, have been found to have amyloid plaques in the brain at autopsy and seemed to have a heightened risk of AD. While we don't have a correlation to a specific virus or a bacterium, some insidious infections, like prion, may be altering the neuro-inflammatory balance. Both of these suggests that post-infectious autoimmune factors, such as viral I-Cubed, may be a contributing cause of AD in some cases.

AD is now thought to exist on a biological and clinical continuum.[3] There are individual differences in rate of cognitive and functional decline, and not all individuals will progress to AD dementia or through the various AD dementia severities during their lifetime. Memory loss is first apparent as episodic forgetfulness that is characterized by diminished recall,[4] which is thought to be caused by the progressive accumulation of extracellular cortical plaques and intracellular neurofibrillary tangles. The plaques contain Aβ proteins, while neurofibrillary tangles show hyperphosphorylated tau proteins. At this early stage there may also be dysfunction of cholinergic neurons of the basal forebrain.[5] Episodic memory loss is followed by the loss of executive function (e.g., impaired planning and anticipation, or failure to multitask), and language and recognition difficulties. Functional impairment is usually first apparent as subtle deficits in complex activities of daily living, including inability to work the telephone, poor financial decision-making, missing routine appointments, and forgetting how to use everyday technology.[6] Complete impairment in basic functioning, such as eating, dressing, and toileting, is generally not apparent until further along the clinical continuum.

Some early signs of AD include simultaneous autoimmune illnesses like arthritis and the presence of inflammatory biomarkers in the blood stream.[7] Patients with progressive neurodegenerative disorders such as AD[8] often also have gastrointestinal health issues.[9] Genetic studies show that AD is a variable disorder that ranges from early onset, or before age 65 years, to a more common late-onset form.[10] Although PNS and ANS symptoms appear to be increased in mild to moderate AD,[11] affected patients may not report them.

My mother had AD, and her earliest symptom, which occurred when she was just 63, was an inability to unlock and open the bathroom door. She then lost the ability to drive because she couldn't put the key in the ignition to start the car. Eventually, she needed assistance just to open the front door. For my family, these small changes were heartbreaking. At the time, I was a medical student, and my wife and I realized that my mother couldn't watch over our young children, because they could run out the door and she wouldn't know what to do or how to anticipate their activity.

TESTING FOR AD

It used to be that AD could only be properly diagnosed on autopsy, yet today we have biomarkers available for detecting preclinical AD determinants, including bloodwork and tests for CSF. These tests can determine if you have the gene and/or the inflammatory buildup, or occurrence of tau protein.

Initial laboratory investigations are focused on evaluating for other causes of brain dysfunction, and a detailed assessment is often needed to exclude other diseases that can cause cognitive issues. Complete blood count, kidney function and electrolytes, liver function tests and ammonia, vitamin B12, thyroid function, urinalysis, and chest x-ray are important initial tests in evaluating the underlying cause of cognitive impairment. Evaluation for infective causes of indolent cognitive impairment including Lyme serology should be considered, whereas more fulminant cases are likely due to viral encephalitis including West Nile virus encephalitis that may worsen with immunosuppression.

In some cases, brain biopsy may be considered, particularly in patients who do not respond to immunotherapy, as it may help exclude other causes (especially infections and tumors), and, if suggestive of an underlying autoimmune issue, may allow more confidence to embark on a regimen of immune modulation. Suspicion of a reversible autoimmune dementia should be heightened when the biopsy shows perivascular lymphocytic (B- or T-cell) infiltrates and gliosis with or without meningeal involvement,[12] but it may also be helpful when it shows another disorder such as sarcoidosis or granulomatous vasculitis. Notwithstanding, it can offer certain proof of AD neuropathology.

A screen for cancer should be conducted in all patients beginning with CTs of the chest, abdomen, and pelvis, and consideration of PET of the body to increase the detection of an early occult or hidden cancer.

TREATMENT OF AD

Current existing therapies for AD have either no or minimal disease modifying benefit. However, new breakthroughs in treatment have hit on the autoimmune components of the disease and may well be a way to thwart the progression. Preclinical studies show the promise of immunotherapy in the prevention of both AD[13] and prion disease.[14] With a central role for Aβ in the hypothetical model of the amyloid cascade, several strategies envision the eradication of Aβ and its downstream targets.[15]

There is a preponderance of evidence that people that are highest risk for AD genetically be placed on anti-inflammatory medication and follow an anti-inflammatory diet. Over the last decade, passive immunization using anti-Aβ antibodies present in IVIg has held great promise as a potential new disease modifying therapy for AD. The principle of passive immunotherapy in AD is to reduce the levels of toxic Aβ species in the brain. Three postulated molecular mechanisms for the benefit of immunoglobulin immunotherapy in AD include the ameliorative effects of increased efflux and disaggregation of Aβ from the brain, the inhibition of Aβ deposition in vicinity of neurons, and slowing of the amyloid cascade. The latter postulates that Aβ aggregation, especially in its toxic form, is the principal insult, which produces neuronal toxicity and triggers downstream signaling events that in turn lead to hyperphosphorylation of tau and development of neurofibrillary tangles. Although IVIg treatment and other immunotherapies do not significantly slow the rate of cognitive decline in patients with AD, treatment with IVIg early in the course of the disease in older adults is theoretically beneficial.

Because of the limited efficacy of current pharmacological therapy and the knowledge that caring for people with AD and dementia requires the involvement of a large number of professionals (e.g., psychologists, occupational therapists, etc.) and caregivers to offer comprehensive and individualized management, research has focused on non-pharmacological treatment to improve function, independence, and quality of life.[16] These interventions encompass a wide range of interventions ranging from environmental interventions to cognitive rehabilitation therapy.[17] They are not necessarily aimed at influencing underlying pathophysiological mechanisms but at maintaining function and meaningful participation in the activities of daily living, as the disease progresses, thus reducing disability and improving quality of life.

One such cognitive therapy is called the Tailored Activity Program,[18] which brings occupational therapists into the patient's home to try to preserve their cognitive abilities and reduce troubling behaviors that can accompany dementia, including repeated questions, wandering, rejecting assistance, and verbal and physical aggression. A pilot study with the Tailored Activity Program[19] showed that at 4 months, intervention caregivers reported reduced frequency of troubling behaviors, specifically for repetitive questioning, greater activity engagement, and ability to keep busy; and fewer episodes of agitation or argumentation that often trigger nursing home placement. These benefits allowed family members to spend fewer daily hours caring for them, and delayed or prevented potentially costly and dehumanizing nursing home placement.

PARSING BETWEEN AD AND ADE

Autoimmune dementias and encephalopathies (ADEs) are complex disorders that lead to symptoms of immune-mediated cognitive deficits that resemble AD, but differ significantly in their presentation and diagnosis. First, with ADEs there is an absence of progressive neurocognitive and behavioral deterioration: the changes come across suddenly. ADE symptoms may occur in the presence of a known cancer, and the presence of a personal or family history of autoimmunity or abnormalities in the brain's medial temporal lobe may also be clues underlying ADE. A total of 35 percent of patients in one series of 46 patients who were initially assigned a neurodegenerative diagnosis such as AD were in fact later diagnosed with ADE and subsequently improved with immunotherapy.[20]

TESTING AND TREATING ADES

The availability of testing is crucial to separate those suffering from AD from those with ADE, who do not have the genetic predisposition or characteristic pathology, though in many ways, ADE can look just like AD. The former appears to account for most cases with dementia with onset of symptoms before 45 years of age,[21] in contrast to AD which affects individuals later in life. Like other autoimmune disorders, ADEs are more common in women, but there is a wide age range of onset and, although most frequent in mid-late adulthood, children and very elderly adults may be affected.[22]

ADE can look like a dementing illness, defined as impairment in two or more of the five cognitive domains (learning and memory, language, executive function, visuospatial skills, and psychomotor function), that interferes with the activities of daily life, not occurring in the setting of delirium or depression, and representing a decline from a prior level of function.[23] Memory loss is a prominent symptom in ADE, but not all cognitive domains may be affected as in AD. The presentation may mimic a subtype of degenerative dementia called frontotemporal dementia, with personality changes, loss of social conduct, and executive dysfunction with preservation of memory.[24]

Assessing for the presence of neural-specific autoantibodies in blood and CSF has become a critical component in the evaluation of dementia, particuarly in the evaluation of suspected ADE to exclude potential infective etiologies; the presence of inflammation gives a clue to an inflammatory/autoimmune cause. However, there are cases of immunotherapy-responsive dementia with positive AD biomarkers. However, there are cases of immunotherapy-responsive dementia with positive AD biomarkers and postmortem neuropathology suggesting that ADE and AD may coexist, and at the least, immunotherapy lessens the associated inflammatory response.[25]

In many cases of autoimmune ADE, brain MRI may be normal. However, PET/MRI reveals useful determinants of tissue metabolism correlated with brain structure. These include medial temporal lobe abnormalities more commonly in patients with autoantibodies to intracellular antigens (IAg) seen in Type I AE. Brain SPECT may also be performed in ADE, but the findings are less well characterized. Electroencephalography is an important component of the evaluation of patients with suspected ADE; however, the findings are generally nonspecific. The most frequent finding is slowing of brain processing speed, which can be diffuse or focal.

High-dose corticosteroids are the most common initial treatment and may serve as a diagnostic test when a diagnosis is uncertain. Repeat cognitive testing after immunotherapy helps document objective improvements. Maintenance immunotherapy such as IVIg therapy is recommended in those at risk for relapse.

Meet Marty

Marty was a 78-year-old man who came to see me complaining of numbness, tingling, and limb pain. He also had lightheadedness and cognitive decline for one year. Neurological examination showed impaired short-term registration, sensory loss in the legs, imbalance, leg weakness, and absent reflexes. Autonomic testing showed orthostatic hypotension. Electrodiagnostic studies showed peripheral demyelinating neuropathy. Skin biopsy for epidermal nerve fiber densities were consistent with a small fiber neuropathy. Left sural nerve biopsy showed a peripheral neuropathy. Blood studies showed an elevated total prostate-specific antigen of 4.6 ng/mL (normal ≤ 4 ng/mL) that suggested prostate cancer. Brain PET showed temporoparietal and frontal lobe brain hypometabolism. Cerebral spinal fluid testing showed no inflammation or infection. Athena Diagnostics (Massachusetts) ADmark analysis was inconclusive for symptomatic AD. To me, this meant that Marty clearly had many of the signs of autoimmunity, which may be causing his AD symptoms. However, a Mayo Clinic autoimmune dementia panel (ENS1) showed elevated titers of serum nicotinic acetylcholine receptor (nAChR) ganglionic antibodies. Circulating nAChR ganglionic antibodies are associated with autonomic failure[26] because they react with a receptor present on autonomic ganglia. The indeterminate biomarkers for AD along with the clinical features of autoimmune autonomic neuropathy, and large and small fiber peripheral neuropathy and circulating nAChR ganglionic antibodies in the blood, defined him as likely having ADE, and not AD.

I started Marty on an IVIg protocol, and in 6 months we saw the stabilization of his condition. He died two years after initiation of treatment. His autopsy showed frequent neuritic plaques and neurofibrillary tangles in the hippocampus, amygdala, and association cortex without microglial nodules or inflammation.[27] There was also a small cancer of the prostate that was confined to the capsule without metastases. Spinal nerve roots and peripheral nerves showed patchy myelin loss. To me, this meant that Marty was the exceptional patient with ADE in life and AD at death, suggesting a continuum of AE in dementia.

The Surprising Link between COVID-19 and I-Cubed

Beginning in late November 2019, a novel, or new, coronavirus was identified in the Wuhan province of China. A coronavirus is named for the shape of the virus, which has surface projections that resemble a corona or halo. The projections are the viral spike proteins that attach to and invade human host cells.

Coronaviruses possess one of the longest single strands of ribonucleic acid (RNA), a staggering thirty thousand base pairs, making it one of the largest genomes in the virus world. In fact, six of the seven known human coronaviruses that cause disease[1] are already widely prevalent. Yet for this severe acute respiratory syndrome (SARS-CoV-2) coronavirus known as "COVID," we are still working out the explanation of its origin and the cause of the 2019 pandemic.[2] What we do know is that its resulting epidemic outbreak on every continent made it the third and most devastating coronavirus pandemic since the SARS outbreak of 2002 in China,[3] followed by the Middle East Respiratory Syndrome[4] a decade later in Saudi Arabia. Researchers believe that the COVID-19 pandemic was not caused by a mutation of either of the other two deadly coronaviruses. One intriguing characteristic that defines this coronavirus is its ability to mutate, which appears to have allowed it to get a foothold in one part of the globe and then move by human travel to other countries.

As I watch the pandemic unfold in real time and witness firsthand the chronic nervous system complaints of COVID Long Haulers, it is clear to me that COVID is one of many infections that trigger an autoimmune response.

It evokes the same I-Cubed playbook of *infection* leading to *immunity*, which leads to *inflammation*, and it is a formidable microbial trigger, just as we saw with Lyme disease or in the relationship between strep infection and PANS. In fact, given the attention that we're paying to COVID right now and the intensity with which we're understanding its subsequent cytokine storm, it is now the best understood of all the I-Cubed disorders and lays the groundwork for understanding all the others in better detail.

Just as we did for other I-Cubed infections, let's figure out exactly what COVID is and how it infects, and affects, the body.

HOW COVID INFECTS THE BODY

A COVID infection generally begins the same way with every patient: after an exposure, the viral spike proteins attach to a human host's angiotensin-converting enzyme 2 (ACE2) receptor, in much the same way a key fits into a lock.[5] However, for the first five to six days after exposure, the COVID spike proteins are invisible to the host, allowing it to evade detection by the host's immune system. During this time, the body isn't aware that the virus is creeping around, but the infective process is completed. This characteristic of evading the immune system, which is the most important evolutionary feature of COVID, has enabled it to effectively spread among large populations.

After the virus enters the human host through the nose, it enters the host's other cells through a series of steps. First, the viral proteins are digested by dissolving enzymes called *cathespins* that fuse the outer cell membranes of the virus and host, allowing it to enter the cells and release its genetic material. This prepares the virus for replication and a continued life cycle in the host, where it translates its RNA material into functioning viral proteins before being released into the bloodstream to travel to other organs. By the time it enters a cell, the body's immune system recognizes it as an intruder, and the alarms go off. Either you have an appropriate immune response and the immune system attacks it and gets rid of it, or you have an inappropriate immune response that leads to continued development and the collateral damage, which is the much talked about *cytokine storm*. For the majority of healthy people with a strong immune system, the virus is killed off quickly. For those who don't have a strong immune system, the virus continues to replicate. In effect, the immune response to COVID is sort of a race to the finish of whether the immune system will win over the virus, or the virus will win over it.

The cytokine storm is produced by the release of inflammatory cytokines, especially interleukins (ILs) and tumor necrosis factor (TNF)-α that direct a wave of immune responses against the coronavirus with massive immediate and long-lasting collateral damage. The host's immune system response to the virus resembles a game of whack-a-mole, as the virus pops up and down, evading capture. Like the game, this novel coronavirus is adept at manipulating the host's immune response by engaging in what appears to be a high-stakes game of hide and seek; for some, the immune system response is overkill.

Not everyone who is infected with COVID experiences a cytokine storm, but those who do will most likely have to be hospitalized. They experience immune-mediated damage of previously healthy tissues, beginning with the lungs. A resulting systemic immune response leads to multiple organ effects, including in the heart causing myocarditis and a heart attack, or in the kidneys with resultant renal failure. One important consequence of the cytokine storm is the increased risk of body-wide clotting and occlusion of veins that results in deep vein thromboses of the limbs and arteries, which can lead to fatal pulmonary clots or emboli that cause blood oxygen to reach potentially fatal levels. What's more, the network of secreted cytokines that fuel this storm communicate directly with the central nervous system (CNS) through receptor channels or indirectly across a disrupted blood–brain barrier, which culminates in inflammatory neural tissue damage. The increased levels of oxidative stress and circulating free radicals in the CNS can lead to pruning of brain neurons and their synapses. The collective insults of the cytokine storm lead to the long-lasting complaints of breathing difficulty, sleep problems, pervasive fatigue, pain, and the neurocognitive and neuropsychiatric disturbances reminiscent of chronic fatigue syndrome.[6]

This autoimmune response raises an important question: Is the disease virulence and lethality related to the virus alone or to the inflammatory response it often creates? The answer lies in the dynamic nature of I-Cubed, which postulates that protective immunity becomes the source of autoimmunity conditioned by the environment and genetic factors.[7] This definition of I-Cubed leads to two plausible deductions in understanding the novel coronavirus. First, COVID is the direct trigger of an autoinflammatory response. Second, the dysregulated immune response that follows the infection prompts other insults in the host that lead to the observed pathologies which may vary among individuals due to their genetics and preexisting illnesses. This is why

I believe that early intervention with the TAPES protocol, including antiviral and immune modulation, especially with intravenous immune globulin (IVIg) therapy, are the best hope of a full recovery in severe cases.

A BETTER UNDERSTANDING OF COVID ANTIBODIES

The interesting thing about comparing the antibody response of Lyme disease and COVID is that everyone would love to have antibodies to COVID, but not to Lyme disease. As happy as you'd be to be protected from COVID by carrying a hefty dose of antibodies, we wouldn't share the same happiness if we're a Lyme patient, or a *Bartonella* patient, or even a *Babesia* patient, unless we could believe that having them meant we really must be infected. The reason is that not all antibodies are the same: it's time for a short lesson in *seroconversion*.

Seroconversion refers to the appearance of different types of antibodies, and in the case of COVID, we are specifically looking for IgM and IgG antibodies in the blood. This term specifically refers to a switch from early IgM antibodies that appear days to a week after the initial COVID infection, to the long-lasting IgG type that are better able to neutralize microbes like the coronavirus. IgG antibodies also become highly protective, making it difficult for someone with plenty of them to develop another COVID infection. We now know that most people who get COVID naturally develop protective IgG antibodies that last at least ninety days. When you get vaccinated, the body responds just like it was infected, but seroconversion is bypassed to immediately create stronger, neutralizing IgG antibodies.

Whether you have antibodies from a natural infection or vaccination, there are several reasons to continue to test for them. First, observing a robust antibody response assures that you have the best protection from another COVID exposure. Second, if antibody levels are no longer detectable, you are no longer protected and it is time for a vaccine booster. Third, if you know that you have an immune-compromising disorder, you may be a candidate for either monthly high-dose (two grams per kilogram body weight) intravenous (IVIg) or low-dose (four hundred milligrams per kilogram) subcutaneous Ig.

THE MOST COMMON COVID SYMPTOMS

COVID symptoms typically appear after an incubation period of about five days following exposure. They are often similar to a mild upper respiratory infection, or the flu, with fatigue, fever, and dry cough. What differentiates COVID is an early loss of smell that occurs in up to 96 percent of cases.

COVID infects olfactory cells lining the nasal cavities where viral loads are high at the onset of infection. From there, COVID travels along tiny nerve fibers to synapses on neurons of the olfactory bulbs before crossing into the CNS, where it invades neuronal brain centers that regulate the conscious appreciation and localization of smell, leaving behind evidence of viral RNA and inflammation.[8]

In 20 percent of cases, the viral infection progresses down the trachea to the lung alveoli lined with epithelial cells, wherein it induces them to undergo a programmed cell death, or *apoptosis*, associated with the autoimmune response of secreting cytokines that cause further localized inflammation. This response has the unfortunate consequence of collateral lung tissue damage[9] leading to bilateral organizing pneumonia.[10] This is the point at which patients are placed on machine ventilation to offset the work of breathing, in order to maintain adequate ventilation and oxygenation.

In severe cases, the virus will disseminate from the lungs to other organs such as the heart, kidney, gastrointestinal tract, and brain, where it causes new areas of damage through direct invasion and a collateral immune-mediated damage to tissues.[11]

WHO IS MOST LIKELY TO SUFFER FROM SERIOUS COVID SYMPTOMS?

The differing manifestations and severity of incident cases often, but not always, reflect an individual's preexisting medical conditions. Your genetics can make you a sitting duck for contracting COVID and potentially suffering more severe illness if you have primary immune deficiency or a secondary immune deficiency disorder due to an autoimmune illness or a cancer, or if you take immune suppressive medication.

There are two types of preexisting risk factors to consider: modifiable and nonmodifiable. The latter are ones that cannot be changed, such as a person's age, ethnicity, and genetics. Modifiable disease risk factors are those that can be altered by adopting healthy body and brain behaviors and instituting medical treatments for reversible disorders.

Investigators at the UK Biobank[12] studied risk factors for the outcome of individuals hospitalized with life-threatening COVID. They found a worse outcome of COVID compared to non-COVID controls in older age unemployed or retired non-white men with the following *modifiable* risks: autoimmune disease, hypertension, diabetes, obesity, low vitamin D level, prescription steroids and statins, cigarette smokers, and those residing in areas with high air pollution. There may be other modifiable risks that come out of research. In the meantime, practice healthy behaviors as outlined in TAPES and seek treatment for modifiable illnesses to avert a deadly outcome.

NEUROLOGIC COVID SYMPTOMS

The neurologic manifestations of COVID are most common after loss of lung function and are noted in more than 80 percent of adult cases. Children younger than 18 years of age account for an estimated 5 percent of reported cases, and the most significant neurological involvement in this age group occurs in about half of cases. These children can develop the potentially fatal childhood disorder *multisystem inflammatory syndrome* (MIS-C), which presents with a combination of any of the following: fatigue, fever, rash, headache, aseptic meningitis, seizures, brain fog, lethargy, and coma.[13] These symptoms may progress even after a course of antiviral therapy[14] due to the cytokine storm.

Neurologic symptoms in adults range from mild headache to seizures, peripheral neuropathy, stroke, demyelinating CNS disease, and encephalopathy. However, those with increased baseline serum cytokine and pro-coagulation markers at the time of hospitalization appear to have the worst prognosis.[15]

Brain insults resulting from the neurotrophic infection, added to the post-infectious autoinflammatory insult of brain cells, can be clinically studied and even prognosticated using high-tech brain scans, notably [18]fluorodeoxy-glucose positron emission tomography (FDG PET) combined with magnetic resonance imaging (MRI) and three-dimensional software (PET/MRI). Together, they differentiate two important effects of COVID: metabolic changes or "under-functioning" and structural damage or lesions. In my study,[16] I found that a surprising 16 percent of cases had unrecognized fatal brainstem encephalitis. We also found compelling evidence showing that COVID targets cortical neurons that localize hyperphosphylated Tau, which is a known driver of neurodegeneration in Alzheimer's disease[17] and bipolar disorder.[18] However, we do not know at present whether COVID survivors will be more likely to suffer from these conditions later in life.

Parsing the cause of neurologic symptoms is not simply an academic undertaking for two important reasons. First, the metabolic changes seen on

FDG PET, especially in the temporal lobe hippocampus, an area that I refer to as the "shock-absorber," lead to brain fog, cognitive loss, depression, and worse psychiatric symptoms. These patients have the best chance of resolving with IVIg, selective serotonin and norepinephrine reuptake inhibitors, and cognitive therapy, whereas demyelination and other structural changes on MRI and the symptoms they cause are typically more pervasive and much slower to resolve, if at all, despite the same treatment.

CHRONIC ILLNESS: THE LONG HAULER OR LONG COVID

The scientific community finally recognizes the propensity of COVID to manifest chronic symptoms long after the acute phase of infection. Although most of these patients prefer to be called "Long Haulers," the National Institutes of Health has adopted the term *Post-Acute-Sequelae of SARS-CoV-2*, or the abbreviation PASC, for those who fail to recover from acute COVID-19 and are persistently symptomatic for more than thirty days with any pattern of tissue injury including the nervous system.[19]

Feedback from web-based international surveys of impacted individuals has now resulted in two online research studies.[20, 21] To date, more than seven thousand Long Hauler respondents have reported an average of fourteen symptoms, often in combination, and frequently including the following neurologic issues:

- Balance difficulty
- Chest tightness
- Cognitive dysfunction
- Coldness
- Dizziness
- Dry cough
- Electric shock sensations
- Excessive early fatigue
- Exertional malaise
- Facial paralysis/pressure/numbness
- Headaches
- Memory complaints
- Muscle aches
- Palpitations

- Shortness of breath
- Sore throat
- Speech and language issues
- Weakness

TREATING COVID

If COVID symptoms do not resolve on their own from an appropriate immune response, a likely course of treatment is one of the therapies approved by the US Food and Drug Administration: remdesivir or a monoclonal antibody cocktail. Both medications stop viral replication. However, they do not convincingly demonstrate clinical benefit in very sick hospitalized patients, perhaps because in later stages of the disease, the autoimmune response of toxic inflammation and coagulopathy plays a greater role in a patient's outcome than viral replication.[22]

I have found that IVIg therapy has an unmistakable benefit for both acute patients and Long Haulers.[23] Treatment with high-dose IVIg therapy administered over four to five consecutive days in the early stages of clinically apparent COVID in small case series[24] and randomized clinical trials[25] was associated with clinical stabilization and reduced mortality. IVIg is also a first-line therapy in two potentially fatal and closely related autoinflammatory childhood disorders encountered early in the COVID-19 lockdown: namely, Kawasaki disease and MIS-C.[26]

I have also found that people who are already taking IVIg are more likely to be asymptomatic or have a milder case of COVID, which may be related to improved surveillance of host immunity or stabilization of the immune system. Baseline low immunoglobulin and albumin levels and increased C-reactive protein, IL-6 levels, and naïve helper T-cells that indicate activation of the adaptive cell immunity also predict who will likely suffer from the cytokine storm,[27] making such patients ideal candidates for early immune modulation with IVIg or other immune modulatory agents.

In an early study to determine the potential IVIg treatment for COVID, I followed[28] one hundred adult patients who received IVIg therapy for the treatment of other I-Cubed illnesses. Among them, we found no new cases of COVID. A follow-up survey found only ten (1 percent) of patients testing positive for COVID, all of whom were mild or asymptomatic. This uncontrolled observation suggests that IVIg therapy may have an important role in COVID prevention especially in vulnerable individuals with autoimmune disorders.

A new in-depth interview analysis is studying the lived experiences of adults recruited online[29] who have taken low- or high-dose IVIg before COVID illness to respectively treat immune deficiency or a neuroimmune (I-Cubed) disorder, and another cohort of subjects with Long COVID and a newly diagnosed neuroimmune disorder. In those already receiving IVIg, their subsequent COVID illness was mild and the established neurological disorder only minimally exacerbated. The cohort with Long COVID neurologic symptoms generally reported improved or reversed CNS and peripheral and autonomic nervous system (PNS, ANS) symptoms after high-dose IVIg.

The lived experiences of these subjects were poignantly expressed in several themes. Among all subjects there was a strong impression of not being believed by doctors about the severity of post-COVID symptoms. Another is that they present as "healthy" in normal tests (blood work, physical exams). Many subjects said they were turned away from hospitals and doctor offices and resorted to substantial self-advocacy and research to find specialists to "dig deeper" into their experiences and symptoms to find answers. Subjects with known autoimmune illness or immune incompetence mentioned that they generally did not test positive for COVID on an initial test but did do so on repeat testing, suggesting that standard diagnostic tests might be flawed or affected by their underlying conditions. IVIg in those already taking it did not appear to be a factor in receiving a positive rapid antigen or polymerase chain reaction (PCR) COVID test. In my study, not all patients experienced side effects or had a reaction to IVIg. However, among those who did, the side effects were more noticeable in the beginning, were milder, and were of shorter duration; in addition, there was evidence of no reactions after a few months of regular treatment.

COVID symptoms that have improved with the use of IVIg therapy include:

- Return of smell
- Return of taste
- Improvement in pain
- Resolution of weakness
- Reduced muscle twitching
- Reduced fatigue

- Improved stamina
- Improved body temperature regulation
- Regrowth of hair/cessation of hair loss
- Improved brain fog
- Improved focus and memory
- Improved psychiatric symptoms
- Improved palpitations

A recent publication[30] provides preliminary guidance in the use of high-dose and low-dose IVIg during COVID. Awaiting the results of future randomized clinical trials, IVIg is indicated in the treatment of PASC with well-recognized stigmata of widespread nervous system involvement, implicating tandem CNS, PNS, and ANS involvement. Other potential uses of IVIg during COVID include the following:

1. High-dose IVIg may be considered in select cases of acute COVID to attenuate the post-infectious autoimmune cytokine storm that may result in PASC.
2. Low-dose IVIg may be considered in vaccinated and especially unvaccinated patients to provide immune support during COVID-related illness.
3. Low-dose IVIg may also be considered in patients with primary and secondary immune deficiency to restore immune competence and protection against COVID exposure.
4. High-dose IVIg may also be considered in patients with primary and secondary immune deficiency who succumb to acute COVID to avert further complications including the cytokine storm and PASC.

The following case illustrates the importance of intensively evaluating post-COVID neurologic complaints, as these patients are suffering and may be candidates for IVIg, which has the capacity, as in other I-Cubed illnesses, to impart sustained improvement.

Meet Tonya

Tonya, a fifty-three-year-old corporate consultant, saw a variety of doctors in the summer of 2020 several months after she tested positive for COVID because of her continued struggles with upper respiratory complaints, loss of taste, erratic pulse and blood pressure readings, fatigue, neuropathic pain, weakness, and brain fog.

Tonya finally came to see me in December 2020, and I found sensory loss to vibration, cold temperature, and pin prick, and weakness in the arms and legs with reduced tendon reflexes. Electrodiagnostic studies showed chronic demyelinating and axonal nerve changes consistent with peripheral neuropathy. Epidermal nerve fiber densities in biopsies of skin were reduced in the thigh and calf, indicative of small fiber neuropathy. Tilt table test showed dysautonomia with a precipitous fall in blood pressure to eighty mmHg and a compensatory increase in the heart rate to 121 beats per minute. FDG PET/ MRI with three-dimensional post-processing showed hypometabolism of the anterior and medial temporal lobes consistent with encephalopathy. Mayo Clinic autoimmune encephalopathy (ENS2) panel showed no autoantibodies. I started her on a high-dose monthly IVIg, and Tonya found steady improvement and was nearly normal when last seen in the summer 2021.

BOX 21.1

SUFFERING FROM PANDEMIC BURNOUT?

Whether you are reading this chapter because you want to know more about COVID or believe that you are a Long Hauler and are wondering when life will return to normal (if ever), you can take solace in knowing that if you are feeling burnout, you are not alone.

Lucy McBride, an internist in Washington, DC, wrote in *The Atlantic*[31] that the symptoms of burnout have become more medical, and less so job-related, explaining it as the work of living through the COVID pandemic. She ascribed feelings of burnout to the accumulated stresses of the pandemic life coupled with entering the non-pandemic life that was left behind. She suggests taking charge of your life again to restore a sense of self-determination, reassessing and simplifying your home life, work, and relationships in accordance with your abilities, and setting realistic expectations.

THE DILEMMA OF VARIANTS

Viruses are constantly mutating because they are under pressure to survive, resulting in variants. Each variant is endowed with genetic characteristics that allow it to spread more easily or make it resistant to treatments or vaccination, compared to the initial wild type. This is because their pathological makeup makes them even more resilient than the original strain and able to bind to host receptor proteins more efficiently. Currently, multiple variants of COVID are circulating globally. As of this writing, there have been four notable CO-VID variants: the UK B.1.1.7 (alpha), the South African B.1.351 (beta), the Brazilian P.1 (gamma), and the Indian B.1.617.2 (delta).

While infections seemed to be vanishing in the United States with vac-cination, recent outbreaks suggest that the numbers are climbing as a result of the more highly contagious delta variant, especially among unvaccinated people and even among the fully and more so non-partially vaccinated people. Effectiveness of one vaccine dose (Pfizer) was far less against delta than for alpha (30 percent versus 48 percent) and only modestly different in those fully vaccinated (88 percent versus 93 percent).[32] While fully vaccinated people are likely to have mild symptoms with a breakthrough infection, those that haven't been vaccinated at all, or who have had only one dose, may be hospi-talized with more severe illness.

A Case of PANDAS Plus COVID: Meet Yanni

The following patient came to me with an exacerbation of a latent neuropsy-chiatric disorder, which reappeared after two different COVID exposures. An eleven-year-old named Yanni had a history of recurrent strep infections and often experienced the behavioral changes associated with PANDAS. Then in March 2020, his whole family, including Yanni, got COVID. While the rest of his family had an easy time recovering, his health continued to go downhill. By November, he became reclusive and afraid of people; he refused to leave the house. Eventually Yanni became violent, smashing out windows, punch-ing, and hurling things at his family.

The following September, he was supposed to return to in-person learn-ing, but it became a daily struggle to get Yanni to leave the house. Something seemed to be attacking his body and mind. One doctor diagnosed him with high-level functioning autism, attention deficit hyperactivity disorder, and depression. He tried different psychiatric medications, but nothing helped.

In February 2021 he came to see me, and we started him on a month of IVIg therapy. This seemed to bring his condition to a standstill until early August, when the delta variant was in full swing; his violent symptoms returned. I asked Yanni's parents to have him retested. The rapid swab test of the nasopharynx was negative; however, the more sensitive polymerase chain reaction test was positive for the delta variant, even though he had no upper respiratory symptoms. I believe that the second COVID infection with the delta variant worsened his underlying PANDAS, and at that point he became PANS because there was no strep infection. Yanni is now back on IVIg treatment and hopefully will end the cycle of recurrent infection.

TAPES IS PART OF THE COVID PROTOCOL

Along with getting vaccinated, wearing masks, and social distancing, the TAPES protocol as outlined in this book will go a long way to ensuring a healthier immune system. Testing can now include both regular COVID and antibody testing. Applying IVIg therapies may have both preventative and therapeutic responses. Participating in stress reduction and other mental health exercises will keep burnout at bay. Eating high-quality foods and participating in regular exercise not only keep the mind and body well-tuned, but enhance immunity. Lastly, surveying your environment for toxins and pollutants will also allow your immune system to focus on beating the infection, rather than being distracted by noxious exposures.

Putting It All Together to Resolve Your Health

At this point you should have a much better understanding of everything you need to do to restore health to your brain and body. You've learned how the autoimmune response intersects with brain function, and how the two can cause otherwise unexplained symptoms. You have learned that there are three major nervous systems that occur and are controlled by the brain: the CNS, PNS, and ANS. You may also have been able to pinpoint and ascribe your symptoms to one or more of them. And at this point, you may have even started on your path of wellness by adopting some of the easiest practices in the TAPES protocol: diet, exercise, detoxification, and many of the suggestions that reduce stress.

As you've seen throughout the book, I-Cubed diseases often cause overlapping involvement of the CNS, PNS and ANS silos. In part, that's because the biological functions of each of these systems interact every single day, sharing the same DNA and HLA genes, and overlapping neural circuits that are highly integrated with respect to their normal functionality and responses to injury. Moreover, it starts and ends with the brain.

Remember, the brain is the seat of the ANS, which originates in the hypothalamus, driving the autonomic system via the hypothalamic-pituitary-adrenal axis, then the pituitary gland, and eventually the adrenal glands which release adrenaline and cortisol in times of stress. The neural connections of the ANS project along pathways descending from the brain stem and spinal cord through a network that connects to the visceral organs including the heart, lungs, intestines, bladder, and so on, where they release the hormones epinephrine, norepinephrine, and acetylcholine, which regulate bodily functions such as heart rate and blood pressure in accordance with your postural needs.

The PNS is so important in maintaining connectivity to our limbs from outgoing and incoming information in the skin, muscles, and joints that are transmitted to and from the brain for conscious control of voluntary movement, balance, and even dancing when we feel good enough. Yet when illness strikes, there can be a colossal meltdown of function, leading to protracted illness. Circumstance such as these can be humiliating and demoralizing, and sometimes unbelievable to doctors, friends, and family who may think the sufferer is looking for extra attention or not trying hard enough to get better.

At the same time the CNS activity in the brain is the beacon of cognitive and neuropsychological functioning, ranging from your normal intellect, to your moods and ability to store, retrieve, and create new memories. This function is located in the temporal lobe and hippocampus, where, when we are healthy individuals, we have the innate ability to regenerate brain cells that may be lost through aging and illness, yet are critical for continued functioning at the highest levels. Antidepressant medications such as SSRIs and SNRIs are like fertilizer for the hippocampus in its ability to enhance neurogenesis and promote neural plasticity.

Each of these nervous system components is also influenced by our inherited genetic blueprint. Our genes not only determine our risk for certain autoimmune conditions like Celiac disease, they reveal an inherent tendency for mental illness leading to anxiety, depression, and even bipolar disease; our ability to be resilient in the face of stress, injury, or infection; and our chances of developing neurodegenerative disorders like Alzheimer's later in life.

Acquired brain insults through I-Cubed, including infection, traumatic brain injury, autoimmune encephalitis, and systemic metabolic storms such as Hashimoto's thyroiditis can all pierce the BBB, inciting autoimmunity and inflammation in the brain, leading to the brain symptoms.

So how do *your* unique brain and body health symptoms show this intricate overlap of function? Compare the symptoms you inserted into the Venn diagram in chapter 5 to the systems and their disturbed function shown in the figure on the next page. With this visualization, you may have a better sense of your illness and be prepared to convey your thoughts and suspicions to your physicians, who can then help you arrive at the right diagnoses and treatments. These are solvable, and treatable, childhood and adult neurological disorders, and by treating them correctly you can have peace of mind and renewed hope that you and your loved ones will get better.

This overlap points to the reason why TAPES works: different tests and treatments are appropriate for different symptoms, and when there is overlap with symptoms, there will be overlap with treatments. The triggers of illness often fall neatly into the categories of infectious, metabolic, traumatic, toxic, genetic, autoimmune, and even cancerous insults, whether singly or in combination. We can best arrive at determining this by looking at blood tests. Further testing to establish the functionality and disease involvement of each category can then be undertaken. The CNS can be evaluated used using a brain MRI alone or fused with PET to analyze brain tissue morphology and metabolism, while SPECT can assess tissue perfusion and the BBB. Testing of the PNS centers on electromyography and nerve conduction studies to analyze large nerve fibers, and epidermal nerve fiber analysis via skin biopsy to assess the density of small nerve fibers. Testing the ANS typically involves a tilt table study.

Understanding the relationship of injury to repair in the nervous system is crucial to my model. Injury due to disease occurs gradually or precipitously depending upon the disease process, while neural repair is an inevitable and unchanging process that relies upon regeneration, neural plasticity, and neurogenesis. Disease injury moves in like a winter storm laying destruction in its path, while road crews show up to clear the debris at their own pace. When injury or "I" equals repair or "R" (viz. I = R), our illness stays the same, not better or worse. However, when injury outstrips repair (I > R), we lose ground and become clinically worse, and vice versa. Obviously the goal is to reduce injury through effective treatments, making R > I. The repair process, when fully in gear and in the absence of ongoing injury, moves the body towards normality. For instance, the PNS and ANS both have a regenerative ability to restore hard-wire connections. Nerve regeneration occurs at a rate of 1 millimeter per day under optimal circumstances. The brain has innate stem cells that lay down new circuits and the capacity to restore the integrity of a disrupted BBB following a disease insult.

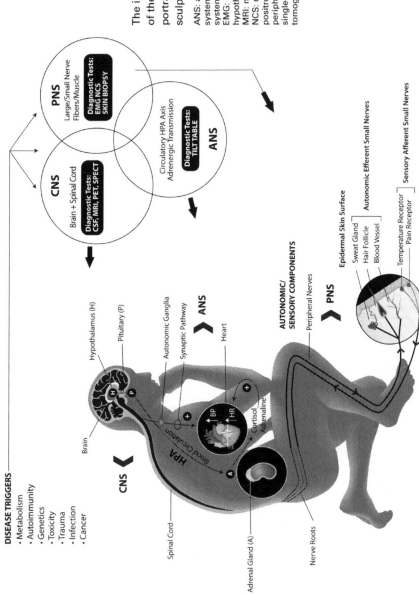

DISEASE TRIGGERS
- Metabolism
- Autoimmunity
- Genetics
- Toxicity
- Trauma
- Infection
- Cancer

PNS
Large/Small Nerve Fibers/Muscle
Diagnostic Tests: EMG NCS SKIN BIOPSY

CNS
Brain + Spinal Cord
Diagnostic Tests: CSF, MRI, PET, SPECT

ANS
Circulatory HPA Axis Adrenergic Transmission
Diagnostic Tests: TILT TABLE

The interconnectedness of the nervous system is portrayed in Auguste Rodin's sculpture of *The Thinker*.

ANS: autonomic nervous system; CNS: central nervous system; CSF: cerebrospinal fluid; EMG: electromyography; HPA: hypothalamic-pituitary-adrenal; MRI: magnetic resonance imaging; NCS: nerve conduction study; PET: positron emission tomography; PNS: peripheral nervous system; SPECT: single-photon emission computed tomography

Hypothalamus (H)
Pituitary (P)
Autonomic Ganglia
Synaptic Pathway
Heart
Brain

CNS

ANS

HPA
Blood Circulation
Cortisol
Adrenaline
BP
HR
A

Spinal Cord
Adrenal Gland (A)
Nerve Roots

AUTONOMIC/ SENSORY COMPONENTS
Peripheral Nerves

PNS

Epidermal Skin Surface
Sweat Gland
Hair Follicle
Blood Vessel
Autonomic Efferent Small Nerves
Temperature Receptor
Pain Receptor
Sensory Afferent Small Nerves

In addressing the underlying autoimmune disorder, the goal is to declare "a truce" in the war being waged upon you by your own immune system. This truce can be effectively orchestrated by removing ongoing disease triggers followed by therapeutically down-regulating T- and B-cell activation in the tri-molecular complex (that includes nascent T cells, the foreign antigen, and the MHC immune playbook with an antigen presenting cell), and recalibrating your immune response through immune therapy. These concepts have been at the center of treating neurological autoimmune disorders for several decades,[1] but only recently have they been actualized and presented to you in this simple format.

To illustrate the model further, you will need to know more about how to recognize repair in response to immunotherapy. The body heals in stages, from "arresting" an illness (meaning there is no further injury on effective treatment), to "remission" status (in which there is no current injury), on the way to a "cure" (when there is no tangible evidence of disease), in both instances, off of medications. An example might be watching a lesion remain stable on brain MRI (arrested, on treatment), and shrink (remission) and eventually disappear (thereby cured) with effective therapy. The decision of whether to use a harsh immunosuppressant agent that reduces both injury and repair, or a gentler immune modulating agent like IVIg, to reduce injury while leaving repair alone, is one I make every day weighing these variables.

Another important consideration is having effective pain management. It turns out the endocannabinoid nervous system of receptors in the brain and on immune cells have receptors ready to battle both pain and inflammation, and are in my mind, better options than opioids because they are not addictive and are equally effective. Legislative efforts to decriminalize these medicines will allow millions of patients to alleviate their pain without stigmatization.

Maintaining an anti-inflammatory lifestyle will address the remainder of your worries for the future. The right foods, the right types of exercise, and consistently practicing methods to reduce stress will help lower inflammation and calm the brain, which is exactly what you need to restore health.

Notes

CHAPTER 1: THE BASICS OF BRAIN HEALTH AND AUTOIMMUNITY

1. Goldsmith CA, Rogers DP. The case for autoimmunity in the etiology of schizophrenia. Pharmacotherapy 2008;28:730–41.

2. Nemeroff CB, Simon JS, Haggerty JJ Jr, et al. Antithyroid antibodies in depressed patients. Am J Psychiatry 1985;142:840–43.

3. Ching KH, Burbelo PD, Carlson PJ, et al. High levels of anti-GAD65 and anti-Ro52 autoantibodies in a patient with major depressive disorder showing psychomotor disturbance. J Neuroimmunol 2010;222:87–89.

4. Twilt M, Benseler SM. Central nervous system vasculitis in adults and children. Handb Clin Neurol 2016;133:283–315.

5. Logigian EI, Johnson KA, Kijewski MF, et al. Reversible cerebral hypoperfusion in Lyme encephalopathy. Neurology 1997;49:1661–70.

6. Coughlin JM, Yang T, Rebman AW, Kortte KB, Du Y, Mathews WB et al. (2018) Imaging Glial Activation in Patients with Post-Treatment Lyme Disease Symptoms: A Pilot Study Using [11C]DPA-713 PET. Journal of Neuroinflammation, 15, 346.

7. Sun Yang, Muo Zhu-Min, Guo Ziu-Ming, et al. An updated role of microRNA-124 in central nervous system disorders: a review. Front Cell Neurosci. https://doi.org/10.3389/fncel.2015.00193.

8. Yeoh SW, Holmes CAN, Saling MM, et al. Depression, fatigue and neurocognitive deficits in chronic hepatitis C. Hepatol Int 2018;Jun 21. doi: 10.1007/s12072-018 -9879-5. [Epub ahead of print].

9. Younger DS. Hashimoto encephalopathy: impact of concussion. World Journal of Neuroscience 2018;8:108–12.

10. Freeman R, Wieling W, Axelrod FB, et al. Consensus statement on the definition of orthostatic hypotension, neurally mediated syncope and the postural tachycardia syndrome. Clin Auton Res 2011;21:69–72.

11. Raj SR. Postural tachycardia syndrome (POTS). Circulation 2013;127:2336–42.

12. Freeman R, Lirofonis V, Farquhar WB, et al. Limb venous compliance in patients with idiopathic orthostatic intolerance and postural tachycardia. J Appl Physiol (1985) 2002;93:636–44.

13. Low PA, Sandroni P, Joyner M, et al. Postural tachycardia syndrome (POTS). J Cardiovasc Electrophysiol 2009;20:352–58.

14. Okamoto LE, Raj SR, Peltier A, et al. Neurohumoral and haemodynamic profile in postural tachycardia and chronic fatigue syndromes. Clin Sci (Lond) 2012;122:183–92.

15. Mathias CJ, Low DA, Iodice V, et al. Postural tachycardia syndrome—current experience and concepts. Nat Rev Neurol 2012;8:22–34.

16. Gazit Y, Nahir AM, Grahame R, et al. Dysautonomia in the joint hypermobility syndrome. Am J Med 2003;115:33–40.

CHAPTER 2: HOW THE BRAIN DEVELOPS

1. Kandel ER, Schwartz JH, Jessell TM. Principles of Neural Science. Amsterdam, Netherlands: Elsevier, 1981.

2. Kandel ER, Schwartz JH, Jessell TM. Siegelbaum SA, Hudspeth AJ. Principles of Neural Science. Fifth edition. McGraw-Hill: New York, 2012.

3. Komisar E, Miner S. Being there: Why prioritizing motherhood in the first three years matters. Tarcher Pergee:New York, 2017.

4. Bruer JT. The myth of the first three years. A new understanding of early brain and lifelong learning. The Free Press:New York, 1999.

5. Nash MJ, Frank DN, Friedman JE. Early microbes modify immune system development and metabolic homeostasist—the "Restaurant" hypothesis revisited. Front Endocrinol (Lausanne) 2017;8:349.

6. Stiles J, Jernigan TL. The basics of brain development. Neuropsychol Rev 2010;20:327–48.

7. Marrus N, Eggebrecht AT, Todorov A, Elison JT, et al. Walking, gross motor development, and brain functional connectivity in infants and toddlers. Cereb Cortex 2018;28:750–63.

8. Dennis EL, Thompson PM. Typical and atypical brain development: a review of neuroimaging studies. Dialogues Clin Neurosci 2013;15:359–84.

9. Sporns O, Tononi G, Kötter R, et al. The human connectome: a structural description of the human brain. PLoS Comput Biol 2005;1:245–51.

10. van den Heuvel MP, Sporns O. Network hubs in the human brain. Trends Cogn Sci 2013;17:683–96.

11. Arnatkevičiūtė A, Fulcher BD, Pocock R, et al. Hub connectivity, neuronal diversity, and gene expression in the caenorhabditis elegans connectome. PLoS Comput Biol 2018;14:1–32.

12. Baptista P, Andrade JP. Adult hippocampal neurogenesis: regulation and possible functional and clinical correlates. Front Neuroanat 2018;12:44.

CHAPTER 3: IS MY PROBLEM NEUROPSYCHIATRIC OR PSYCHIATRIC?

1. Patterson DC, Grelsamer RP. Approach to the patient with disproportionate pain. Bull Hosp Joint Dis (2013) 2018 Jun;76(2):123–32.

2. Vigo D, Thornicroft G, Atun R. Estimating the true global burden of mental illness. The Lancet Psychiatry 2016;3:171–78.

3. Najjar S, Steiner J, Najjar A, et al. A clinical approach to new-onset psychosis associated with immune dysregulation: the concept of autoimmune psychosis. J Neuroinflammation 2018;15:40.

4. Najjar S, Pahlajani S, De Sanctis V, et al. Neurovascular unit dysfunction and blood-brain barrier hyperpermeability contribute to schizophrenia neurobiology: a theoretical integration of clinical and experimental evidence. Front Psychiatry 2017;8:83.

5. Benros ME, Mortensen PB, Eaton WW. Autoimmune diseases and infections as risk factors for schizophrenia. Ann N Y Acad Sci 2012;1262:56–66.

6. Younger DS. Epidemiology of childhood and adult mental illness. Neurol Clin 2016;34:1023–33.

7. Younger DS. Epidemiology of childhood and adult mental illness. Neurol Clin 2016;34:1023–33.

8. Younger DS. Epidemiology of childhood mental illness: a review of U.S. surveillance data and the literature. World Journal of Neuroscience 2017;7:48–54.

9. Rolls ET. Limbic systems for emotion and for memory, but no single limbic system. Cortex 2015;62:119–57.

10. Campbell S, MacQueen G. The role of the hippocampus in the pathophysiology of major depression. Journal of Psychiatry and Neuroscience 2004;29:417–26.

11. MacQueen GM, Campbell S, McEwen BS, et al. Course of illness, hippocampal function, and hippocampal volume in major depression. Proc Natl Acad Sci USA 2003;100:1387–92.

12. Younger DS. Autoimmune encephalitides. World Journal of Neuroscience 2017;7:327–61.

13. Gilbertson MW, Shenton ME, Ciszewski A, et al. Smaller hippocampal volume predicts pathologic vulnerability to psychological trauma. Nat Neurosci 2002;5:1242–47.

14. Metyas SK, Solyman JS, Arkfeld DG. Inflammatory fibromyalgia: is it real? Curr Rheumatol Rev 2015;11:15–17.

CHAPTER 4: OWN YOUR GENETICS

1. Lu G, Zhang M, Wang J, et al. Epigenetic regulation of myelination in health and disease. Eur J Neurosci 2019 Jan 11. doi: 10.1111/ejn.14337. [Epub ahead of print]

2. Khan FA, Al-Jameil N, Khan MF, et al. Thyroid dysfunction: an autoimmune aspect. Int J Clin Exp Med 2015;8:6677–81.

3. Fredericks DN, Relman DA. Localization of *Tropheryma whippelii* rRNA in tissues from patients with Whipple's disease. J Infect Dis 2001;183:1229–37.

4. Panegyres PK. Diagnosis and management of Whipple's disease of the brain. Pract Neurol 2008;8:311–17.

5. Relman DA, Schmidt TM, MacDermott RP, et al. Identification of the uncultured bacillus of Whipple's disease. N Engl J Med 1992;327:293–301.

6. Gershon MD. The Second Brain. New York: HarperCollins Publishers, 1998.

7. Burns AJ, Goldstein AM, Newgreen DF, et al. White paper on guidelines concerning enteric nervous system stem cell therapy for enteric neuropathies. Developmental Biology 2016;417:229–51.

8. Furness JB, Callaghan BP, Rivera LR, Cho HJ. The enteric nervous system and gastrointestinal innervation: integrated local and central control. Adv Exp Med Biol 2014;817:39–71.

9. Clevers H. The intestinal crypt, a prototype stem cell compartment. Cell 2013;154:274–84.

10. Turner JR. Intestinal mucosal barrier function in health and disease. Nat Rev Immunol 2009;9:799–809.

11. Forsythe P, Bienenstock J, Kunze WA. Vagal pathways for microbiome–brain–gut axis communication. Adv Exp Med Biol 2014;817:115–33.

12. Rush AJ, George MS, Sackeim HA, et al. Vagus nerve stimulation (VNS) for treatment-resistant depressions: a multicenter study. Biol Psychiatry 2000;47: 276–86.

13. Klingelhoefer L, Reichmann H. Pathogenesis of Parkinson disease—the gut–brain axis and environmental factors. Nat Rev Neurol 2015;11:625–36.

14. Gershon MD. Serotonin is a sword and a shield of the bowel: serotonin plays offense and defense. Trans Am Clin Climatol Assoc 2012;123:268–80.

15. Alivisator AP, Blaser MJ, Brodie EL, et al. A unified initiative to harness Earth's microbiomes. Science 2015;350:507–08.

16. Dubilier N, McFall-Ngai M, Zhao L. Create a global microbiome effort. Nature 2015;526:631–34.

17. Gur TL, Worly BL, Bailey MT. Stress and the commensal microbiota: importance in parturition and infant neurodevelopment. Front Psychiatry 2015;6:5.

18. Barker DJ, Osmond C. Infant mortality, childhood nutrition, and ischaemic heart disease in England and Wales. Lancet 1986;1:1077–81.

19. Bale TL, Baram TZ, Brown AS, et al. Early life programming and neurodevelopmental disorders. Biol Psychiatry 2010;68:314–19.

20. Ulrich-Lai YM, Herman JP. Neural regulation of endocrine and autonomic stress responses. Nat Rev Neurosci 2009;10(6):397.

21. Aguilera G. HPA axis responsiveness to stress: implications for healthy aging. Exp Gerontol 2011;46(2–3):90.

22. http://www.rccxandillness.com/.

23. Chen W, Xu Z, Nishitani M, et al. Complement component 4 copy number variation and CYP21A2 genotype associations in patients with congenital adrenal hyperplasia due to 21-hydroxylase deficiency. Human Genetics 2012;131:1889–94.

CHAPTER 5: *TEST* FOR AN AUTOIMMUNE DISTURBANCE

1. Tagge CA, Fisher AM, Minaeva OV, et al. Concussion, microvascular injury, and early tauopathy in young athletes after impact head injury and an impact concussion mouse model. Brain 2018;141:422–58.

2. Adapted from, Younger DS. Sports-related concussion in school-age children. World Journal of Neuroscience 2018;8:10–31.

3. Coughlin JM, Yang T, Rebman AW, et al. Imaging Glial Activation in Patients with Post-Treatment Lyme Disease Symptoms: A Pilot Study Using [11C]DPA-713 PET. Journal of Neuroinflammation 2018; 15:346.

4. Younger DS. Serial Brain Positron Emission Tomography Fused to Magnetic Resonance Imaging in Post-Infectious and Autoantibody-Associated Autoimmune Encephalitis. World Journal of Neuroscience 2019; 9:153–156.

CHAPTER 6: *APPLY* IMMUNE-MODULATORY AND PAIN THERAPY

1. https://consultqd.clevelandclinic.org/immune-modulatory-therapy-can-be-right-choice-when-surgery-is-not-indicated-in-rasmussen-epilepsy/.

2. Zuizewind CA, van Kessel P, Kramer CM, et al. Home-based treatment with immunoglobulins: an evaluation from the perspective of patients and healthcare professionals. J Clin Immunol 2018;38(8):876–85.

3. https://www.fda.gov/biologicsbloodvaccines/bloodbloodproducts/approved products/licensedproductsblas/fractionatedplasmaproducts/ucm133691.htm.

4. Bakkers M, Faber CG, Hoeijmakers JGJ, et al. Small fibers, large impact: quality of life in small-fiber neuropathy. Muscle Nerve 2014;49:329–36.

5. Hill KP, Palastro MD, Johnson B, et al. Cannabis and pain: a clinical review. Cannabis and Cannabinoid Research 2017;2:1.

6. Vos T, Flaxman AD, Naghavi M, et al. Years lived with disability (YLDs) for 1160 sequelae of 289 diseases and injuries 1990-2010: a systematic analysis for the Global Burden of Disease Study 2010. Lancet 2012;380:2163–96.

7. Moore A, Derry S, Eccleston C, et al. Expect analgesic failure, pursue analgesic success. BMJ 2013;346:2690.

8. Pizzo PA, Clark NM. Alleviating suffering 101—pain relief in the United States. N Engl J Med 2012;367:197–98.

9. Velander JR. Suboxone: rationale, science, misconceptions. Ochsner J 2018;18:23–29.

10. Dowell D, Haegrich TH, Chou R. CDC guidelines for prescribing opioids for chronic pain-United States, 2016. MMWR Recomm Rep 2016;65:1–48.

11. Baker DW. History of the Joint Commission pain standards: lessons for today's prescription opioid epidemic. JAMA 2017;317:1117–18.

12. Guindon J, Hohmann AG. The endocannabinoid system and pain. CNS & Neurological Disorders Drug Targets 2009;8:403–29.

13. Lee MC, Ploner M, Wiech K, et al. Amygdala activity contributes to the dissociative effect of cannabis on pain perception. Pain 2013;134:123–34.

14. Zhang J, Echeverry S, Lim TK, et al. Can modulating inflammatory response be a good strategy to treat neuropathic pain? Current Pharmaceutical Design 2015;21:831–39.

15. Koppel BS, Brust JCM, Fife T, et al. Systematic review: efficacy and safety of medical marijuana in selected neurologic disorders report of the Guideline Development Subcommittee of the American Academy of Neurology. Neurology 2014;82:1556–63.

16. Aviram J, Samuelly-Leichtag G. Efficacy of cannabis-based medicines for pain management: a systematic review and meta-analysis of randomized controlled trials. Pain Physician 2017;20:E755–E796.

17. Younger DS. A preliminary cost-effectiveness analysis of the treatment of chronic pain in sickle cell disease with medical cannabis. HPAM 823 Health Policy Analysis Methods. December 13, 2018; 1–16.

18. Haroutounian S, Ratz Y, Ginosar Y, et al. The effect of medicinal cannabis on pain and quality-of-life outcomes in chronic pain: a prospective open-label study. Clin J Pain 2016;32:1036–43.

CHAPTER 7: *PARTICIPATE* IN THERAPIES THAT ADDRESS STRESS AND MENTAL HEALTH CONCERNS

1. Miller MW, Maniates H, Wolf EJ, et al. CRP polymorphisms and DNA methylation of the AIM2 gene influence associations between trauma exposure, PTSD, and C-reactive protein. Brain Behav Immun 2017;67:194–202.

2. Passos IC, Vasconcelos-Moreno MP, Costa LG, Kunz M, Brietzke E, Quevedo J, Salum G, Magalhaes PV, Kapczinski F, Kauer-Sant'Anna M. Inflammatory markers in post-traumatic stress disorder: a systematic review, meta-analysis, and meta-regression. Lancet Psychiatry 2015;2:1002-12.

3. Breen MS, Maihofer AX, Glatt SJ, et al. Gene networks specific for innate immunity define post-traumatic stress disorder. Mol Psychiatry 2015;20:1538-45.

4. Luders E, Toga AW, Lepore N, et al. The underlying anatomical correlates of long-term meditation: larger hippocampal and frontal volumes of gray natter. NeuroImage 2009;45(3):672-78.

5. Arden R, Chavez RS, Grazioplene R, et al. Neuroimaging creativity: a psychometric view. Behav Brain Res 2010;214:143-56.

6. Roth, Bob. Strength in Stillness: The Power of Transcendental Meditation. Simon & Schuster: New York, 2018.

7. Hernandez SE, Suero J, Rubia K, et al. Monitoring the neural activity of the state of mental silence while practicing Sahaja yoga meditation. Journal of Alternative and Complementary Medicine 2015;21(3):175-79.

8. Dodich A, Zollo M, Crespi C, et al. Short-term Sahaja Yoga meditation training modulates brain structure and spontaneous activity in the executive control network. Brain Behav 2018;9(1):e01159.

9. Williams JMG, Kabat-Zinn J. Mindfulness: diverse perspectives on its meaning, origins, and multiple applications at the intersection of science and Dharma. Contemp Buddhism 2011;12:1-18.

10. Kabat-Zinn J. Full Catastrophe Living: The Program of the Stress Reduction Clinic at the University of Massachusetts Medical Center. New York, NY: Hyperion, 1990.

11. Segal ZV, Williams JM, Teasdale JD. Mindfulness-based Cognitive Therapy for Depression: A New Approach to Preventing Relapse. New York, NY: Guilford Press, 2002.

12. Kuyken W, Hayes R, Barrett B, Byng R, Dalgleish T, Kessler D, et al. Effectiveness and cost-effectiveness of mindfulness-based cognitive therapy compared with maintenance antidepressant treatment in the prevention of depressive relapse or recurrence (PREVENT): a randomised controlled trial. Lancet 2015;386:63-73.

13. Teasdale JD. Emotional processing, three modes of mind and the prevention of relapse in depression. Behav Res Ther 1999;37(Suppl. 1):S53-S77.

14. Nolen-Hoeksema S. Responses to depression and their effects on the duration of depressive episodes. J Abnorm Psychol 1991;100:569–82.

15. Jha AP, Stanley EA, Kiyonagaet A, al. Examining the protective effects of mindfulness training on working memory capacity and affective experience. Emotion 2010;10(1):54–64.

16. Hölzel BK, Carmody J, Vangel M, et al. Mindfulness practice leads to increases in regional brain gray matter density. Psychiatry Research: Neuroimaging 2011;191(1):36–43.

17. Kim ES, Hagan KA, Grodstein F, et al. Optimism and cause-specific mortality: a prospective cohort study. Am J Epidemiol 2016;185(1):21–29.

18. Ikeda A, Schwartz J, Peters JL, et al. Optimism in relation to inflammation and endothelial dysfunction in older men: the VA Normative Aging Study. Psychosom Med 2011;73(8):664–71.

19. Hingle MD, Wertheim BC, Tindle HA, et al. Optimism and diet quality in the Women's Health Initiative. J Acad Nutr Diet 2014;114(7):1036–45.

20. Tan L, Wang M.-J, Modini M, et al. Preventing the development of depression at work: a systematic review and meta-analysis of universal interventions in the workplace. MBC Medicine 2014;12:74.

21. Deady M, Choi I, Calvo R, et al. eHealth interventions for the prevention of depression and anxiety in the general population: a systematic review and meta-analysis. BMC Psychiatry 2017;17.

22. Gadomski AM, Scribani MB, Krupa N, et al. Pet dogs and children's health: opportunities for chronic disease prevention? Prev Chronic Dis 2015;12:E205.

23. Beetz A, Uvnäs-Moberg K, Julius H, Kotrschal K. Psychosocial and psychophysiological effects of human-animal interactions: the possible role of oxytocin. Front Psychol 2012;3:234.

24. McNicholas J, Collis GM. Children's representations of pets in their social networks. Child Care Health Dev 2001;27(3):279–94.

25. Camp MM. The use of service dogs as an adaptive strategy: a qualitative study. Am J Occup Ther 2001;55:509–17.

26. Burns, DD. Feeling Good: The New Mood Therapy. New York: HarperCollins, 2000.

27. Beck, AT. Depression: Causes and Treatment. Philadelphia: University of Pennsylvania Press, 1972.

28. Hayes SC, Luoma JB, Bond FW, et al. Acceptance and commitment therapy: model, processes and outcomes. Behav Res Ther 2006;44:1–25.

29. Bach P, Hayes SC. The use of acceptance and commitment therapy to prevent the rehospitalization of psychotic patients: a randomized controlled trial. J Consult Clin Psychol 2002;70:1129–39.

30. Wilson KG, Dufrene T. Things Might go Terribly, Horribly Wrong. A Guide to Life Liberated from Anxiety. New Harbinger: Oakland CA, 2010.

31. McMain SF, Chapman AL, Kuo JR, et al. The effectiveness of 6 versus 12-months of dialectical behaviour therapy for borderline personality disorder: the feasibility of a shorter treatment and evaluating responses (FASTER) trial protocol. BMC Psychiatry 2018;18:230.

32. National Center for Education Statistics (NCES). Enrollment Rates of 18- to 24-year-olds in Degree-granting Institutions, by Level of Institution and Sex and Race/Ethnicity of Student: 1967 through 2012. Washington, DC: NCES; 2013. Available at: https://nces.ed.gov/programs/digest/d13/tables/dt13_302.60.asp.

33. Presley CA, Meilman PW, Leichliter JS. College factors that influence drinking. Journal of Studies on Alcohol Supplement. 2002;14:82–90.

34. Alcoholics Anonymous. Fourth Edition, 2001. Alcoholics Anonymous World Services, Inc. New York City.

CHAPTER 8: *EAT AND EXERCISE* TO RESTORE BRAIN HEALTH AND RESET THE IMMUNE SYSTEM

1. Alam R, Abdolmaleky HM, Zhou JR. Microbiome, inflammation, epigenetic alterations, and mental diseases. Am J Med Genet B Neuropsychiatr Genet 2017;174(6):651–60.

2. Chrysohoou C, Panagiotakos DB, Pitsavos C, Das UN, Stefanadis C., Adherence to the Mediterranean diet attenuates inflammation and coagulation process in healthy adults: the ATTICA Study. J Am Coll Cardiol 2004;44(1):152–58.

3. Gómez-Pinilla F. Brain foods: the effects of nutrients on brain function. Nat Rev Neurosci 2008;9(7):568–78.

4. Morris MC, Tangney CC, Wang Y, Sacks FM, Barnes LL, Bennett DA, Aggarwal NT. MIND diet slows cognitive decline with aging. Alzheimer's Dement 2015;11(9):1015–22.

5. Morris MC, Tangney CC, Wang Y, Sacks FM, Bennett DA, Aggarwal NT. MIND diet associated with reduced incidence of Alzheimer's disease. Alzheimer's Dementia 2015;11(9):1007–14.

6. Martinez-Gonzalez MA, Sanchez-Tainta A, Corella D, Salas-Salvado J, Ros E, Aros F, et al. A provegetarian food pattern and reduction in total mortality in the Prevencion con Dieta Mediterranea (PREDIMED) study. Am J Clin Nutr 2014;100(Suppl 1):320S–8S.

7. https://www.healthline.com/nutrition/mind-diet#section1.

8. Hooper L, Martin N, Abdelhamid A, Davey SG. Reduction in saturated fat intake for cardiovascular disease. Cochrane Database Syst Rev 2015;6:CD011737.

9. Chianese R, Coccurello R, Viggiano A, et al. Impact of dietary fats on brain functions. Curr Neuropharmacol 2018;16(7):1059–85.

10. Serhan CN. Lipoxins and aspirin-triggered 15-epi-lipoxins are the first lipid mediators of endogenous anti-inflammation and resolution. Prostaglandins Leukot. Essent Fatty Acids 2005;73(3-4):141–62.

11. Bazinet RP, Layé S. Polyunsaturated fatty acids and their metabolites in brain function and disease. Nat Rev Neurosci 2014;15(12):771–85.

12. Barnard ND, Bunner AE, Agarwal U. Saturated and trans fats and dementia: a systematic review. Neurobiol Aging 2014;35(Suppl. 2):S65–S73.

13. Dyall SC. Long-chain omega-3 fatty acids and the brain: a review of the independent and shared effects of EPA, DPA and DHA. Frontiers in Aging Neuroscience 2015;7:52.

14. Ehninger D, Kempermann G. Neurogenesis in the adult hippocampus. Cell Tissue Res 2008;331:243–50.

15. Smith BD. The Emergence of Agriculture. New York: Scientific American Library, 1995.

16. Elliott P. Production of Sugar in the United States and Foreign Countries. Washington, DC: Government Printing Office, 1917.

17. US Department of Agriculture. U.S. per capita caloric sweeteners estimated deliveries for domestic food and beverage use, by calendar year. In Economic Research Service; 2014.

18. Ervin RB. Prevalence of Metabolic Syndrome among Adults 20 Years of Age and Over, by Sex, Age, Race and Ethnicity, and Body Mass Index: United States, 2003–

2006. Hyattsville, MD: U.S. Dept. of Health and Human Services, Centers for Disease Control and Prevention, National Center for Health Statistics, 2009.

19. Schnack LL, Romani AMP. The metabolic syndrome and the relevance of nutrients for its onset. Recent Pat Biotechnol 2017;11:101–19.

20. Lutter M, Nestler EJ. Homeostatic and hedonic signals interact in the regulation of food intake. J Nutr 2009;139:629–32.

21. Gullo S. The Thin Commandments Diet. The 10 No-Fail Strategies for Permanent Weight Loss. New York: Rodale, 2008.

22. Bisht B, Darling WG, Grossmann RE, et al. A multimodal intervention for patients with secondary progressive multiple sclerosis: feasibility and effect on fatigue. Journal of Alternative and Complementary Medicine 2014;20(5):347–55.

23. Perlmutter D. Grain Brain: The Surprising Truth about Wheat, Carbs, and Sugar—Your Brain's Silent Killers. New York: Little Brown Spark, 2018;
    Perlmutter D. The Better Brain Book: The Best Tool for Improving Memory and Sharpness and Preventing Aging of the Brain. New York: Riverhead, 2005.

24. O'Bryan T, The Autoimmune Fix. How to Stop the Hidden Autoimmune Damage That Keeps You Sick, Fat, and Tired Before It Turns Into Disease. New York: Rodale Books, 2016.

25. Voss MW, Vivar C, Kramer AF, van Praag H. Bridging animal and human models of exercise-induced brain plasticity. Trends Cogn Sci 2013;17:525–44.

26. Liu F, Sulpizio S, Kornpetpanee S, Job R. It takes biking to learn: physical activity improves learning a second language. PLOS One 2017;12(5). doi:10.1371/journal.pone.0177624.

27. Larson EB, Wang L, Bowen JD, McCormick WC, Teri L, Crane P, Kukull W. Exercise is associated with reduced risk for incident dementia among persons 65 years of age and older. Ann Intern Med 2006;144:73–81.

28. Schuch FB, Vancampfort D, Firth J, Rosenbaum S, Ward PB, Silva ES, Hallgren M, Ponce De Leon A, Dunn AL, Deslandes AC, Fleck MP, Carvalho AF, Stubbs B. Physical activity and incident depression: a meta-analysis of prospective cohort studies. Am J Psychiatry 2018;175(7):631–48.

29. Choi KW, Chen C, Stein MB, et al. Assessment of bidirectional relationships between physical activity and depression among adults: a 2-sample Mendelian

randomization study. JAMA Psychiatry. Published online January 23, 2019. doi:10.1001/jamapsychiatry.2018.4175.

30. Yang MN, Clements-Nolle K, Parrish B, Yang W. Adolescent concussion and mental health outcomes: a population-based study. American Journal of Health Behavior 2019;43(2):258–65.

31. Broom DR, Miyashita M, Wasse LK. Acute effect of exercise intensity and duration on acylated ghrelin and hunger in men. J Endocrinol 2017;232(3):411–42.

32. Carter SE, Draijer, Holder SM, Brown L, Thijssen DHJ, Hopkins ND. Regular walking breaks prevent the decline in cerebral blood flow associated with prolonged sitting. J Appl Physiol 1985 2018 Jun 7. doi: 10.1152/japplphysiol.00310.2018. [Epub ahead of print].

33. Saint-Maurice PF, Coughlan D, Kelly SP, Keadle SK, Cook MB, Carlson SA, Fulton JE, Matthews CE. Association of leisure-time physical activity across the adult life course with all-cause and cause-specific mortality. JAMA Netw Open 2019;2(3):e190355.

34. Richardson C, Jull P, Hodges J. Therapeutic exercise for spinal segmental stabilization in low back pain: scientific basis and clinical approach. J Can Chiropr Assoc 2000;44:125.

35. Cugliari G, Boccia G. Core muscle activation in suspension training exercises. J Hum Kinet 2017;56:61–71.

36. Field T. Tai Chi research review. Complement Ther Clin Pract 2011;17:141–46.

37. Wei GX, Xu T, Fan FM, et al. Can Taichi reshape the brain? A brain morphometry study. PLoS One 2013;8:e61038.

CHAPTER 9: *SURVEY* YOUR ENVIRONMENT FOR TOXIC EXPOSURES

1. Siblerud RL, Motl J, Kienholz E. Psychometric evidence that mercury from silver dental fillings may be an etiological factor in depression, excessive anger, and anxiety. Psychological Reports 1994;74(1):67–80.

2. Andersen A, Ellingsen DG, Morland T, et al. A neurological and neurophysiological study of chloralkali workers previously exposed to mercury vapour. Acta Neurologica Scandinavica 1993;88(6):427–33.

3. Jusko TA, Henderson Jr CA, Lanphear BP, Cory-Slechta DA, Parsons PJ, Canfield RL. Blood lead concentrations <10 microg/dL and child intelligence at 6 years of age. Environ Health Perspect 2008;116(2):243–48.

4. Canfield RL, Gendle MH, Cory-Slechta DA. Impaired neuropsychological functioning in lead-exposed children. Dev Neuropsychol 2004;26(1):513–40.

5. Kordas K, Canfield RL, López P, Rosado JL, Vargas GG, Cebrián ME, Rico JA, Ronquillo D, Stoltzfus RJ. Deficits in cognitive function and achievement in Mexican first-graders with low blood lead concentrations. Environ Res 2006;100(3):371–86.

6. Wasserman GA, Staghezza-Jaramillo B, Shrout P, Popovac D, Graziano J. The effect of lead exposure on behavior problems in preschool children. Am J Public Health 1998;88(3):481–86.

7. Bellinger DC, Needleman HL. Intellectual impairment and blood lead levels. N Engl J Med 2003;349:500–02.

8. Schafer D, Lehrman E, Kautzman A, et al. Microglia sculpt postnatal neural circuits in an activity and complement-dependent manner. Neuron 2012;74:691–705.

9. Schinder AF, Gage FH. A hypothesis about the role of adult neurogenesis in hippocampal function. Physiology 2004;9:253–61.

10. Jessberger S, Clark RE, Broadbent NJ, et al. Dentate gyrus-specific knockdown of adult neurogenesis impairs spatial and object recognition memory in adult rats. Learning & Memory 2009;16:147–54.

11. Curtis L, Lieberman A. Adverse health effects of indoor molds. Journal of Nutritional and Environmental Medicine 2004;14(3):261–74.

12. Park J-H, Cox-Ganser JM, Kreiss K, et al. Hydrophilic fungi and ergosterol associated with respiratory illness in a water-damaged building. Environ Health Perspec 2008;116(1):45–50.

13. Mustonen K, Karvonen AM, Kirjavainen P, et al. 2015. Moisture damage in home associates with systemic inflammation in children. Indoor Air 2016;26(3):439–47.

14. Commonwealth of Massachusetts. Special Legislative Committee on Indoor Air Pollution, Indoor Air Pollution in Massachusetts. April 1989.

15. Baughman RP, Culver DA, Judson MA. A concise review of pulmonary sarcoidosis. American Journal of Respiratory and Critical Care Medicine 2011;183(5):573–81.

16. Rea WJ, Pan Y, Griffiths B. The treatment of patients with mycotoxin-induced disease. Toxicology and Industrial Health 2009;25(9-10):711–14.

17. Griffiths BB, Rea, WJ, Griffiths B, and Pan Y. The role of the T lymphocytic cell cycle and an autogenous lymphocytic factor in clinical medicine. Cytobios 1998;93:49–66.

18. https://www.ewg.org/research/ewgs-good-seafood-guide/executive-summary.

19. Zhai Q, Narbad A, Chen W. Dietary strategies for the treatment of cadmium and lead toxicity. Nutrients 2015;7(1):552–71.

20. Fox M. Nutritional influences on metal toxicity: cadmium as a model toxic element. Environ Health Perspect 1979;29:95–104.

21. Reddy SY, Pullakhandam R, Kumar BD. Thiamine reduces tissue lead levels in rats: mechanism of interaction. Biometals 2010;23:247–53.

22. Tandon SK, Flora S, Singh S. Influence of pyridoxine (vitamin B6) on lead intoxication in rats. Ind Health 1987;25:93–96.

23. Monachese M, Burton JP, Reid G. Bioremediation and tolerance of humans to heavy metals through microbial processes: a potential role for probiotics? Appl Environ Microbiol 2012;78:6397–404.

24. Sathaye S, Bagul Y, Gupta S, et al. Hepatoprotective effects of aqueous leaf extract and crude isolates of Murraya koenigii against in vitro ethanol-induced hepatotoxicity model. Exp Toxicol Pathol 2011;63:587–91.

25. Jankovic I, Sybesma W, Phothirath P, et al. Application of probiotics in food products—challenges and new approaches. Curr Opin Biotechnol 2010;21:175–81.

26. Halttunen T, Collado M, El-Nezami H, et al. Combining strains of lactic acid bacteria may reduce their toxin and heavy metal removal efficiency from aqueous solution. Lett Appl Microbiol 2008;46:160–65.

27. Crinnion W. Components of practical clinical detox programs—sauna as a therapeutic tool. Alternative Therapies in Health and Medicine 2007;13(2):S154–S156.

CHAPTER 10: DEVELOPMENTAL DISORDERS AFFECTING CHILDREN AND TEENS

1. Bailey A, Phillips W, Rutter M. Autism: towards an integration of clinical, genetic, neuropsychological, and neurobiological perspectives. J Child Psychol Psychiat 1996;37:89–126.

2. Wakefield AJ, Murch SH, Anthony A, et al. Ileal-lymphoid-nodular hyperplasia, non-specific colitis, and pervasive developmental disorder in children. Lancet 1998;351:637–41.

3. Wakefield AJ, Anthony A, Schepelmann S, et al. Persistent measles virus infection and immunodeficiency in children with autism, ileo-colonic lymphoid nodular hyperplasia and non-specific colitis. Gut 1998;42(Suppl 1):A86.

4. Levy SE, Souders MC, Ittenbach RF, et al. Relationship of dietary intake to gastrointestinal symptoms in children with autistic spectrum disorders. Biol Psychiatry 2007;61(4):492–97.

5. Campbell DB, Sutcliffe JS, Ebert PJ, et al. A genetic variant that disrupts MET transcription is associated with autism. Proc Natl Acad Sci USA 2006;103(45):16834–39.

6. Onore C, Careaga M, Ashwood P. The role of immune dysfunction in the pathophysiology of autism. Brain Behav Immun 2012;26(3):383–92.

7. Hornig M. The role of microbes and autoimmunity in the pathogenesis of neuropsychiatric illness. Curr Opin Rheumatol 2013;25(4):488–795.

8. Williams BL, Hornig M, Buie T, et al. Impaired carbohydrate digestion and transport and mucosal dysbiosis in the intestines of children with autism and gastrointestinal disturbances. PLoS One 2011;6(9):e24585.

9. Singh VK, Singh EA, Warren RP. Hyperserotoninemia and serotonin receptor antibodies in children with autism but not mental retardation. Biol Psychiatry 1997;41(6):753–55.

10. Marler S, Ferguson BJ, Lee EB, Peters B, Williams KC, McDonnell E, Macklin EA, Levitt P, Gillespie CH, Anderson GM, Margolis KG, Beversdorf DQ, Veenstra-VanderWeele J. Brief report: whole blood serotonin levels and gastrointestinal symptoms in autism spectrum disorder. J Autism Dev Disord 2016;46:1124–30.

11. Matondo RB, Punt C, Homberg J, Toussaint MJ, Kisjes R, Korporaal SJ, Akkerman JW, Cuppen E, de Bruin A. Deletion of the serotonin transporter in rats disturbs serotonin homeostasis without impairing liver regeneration. Am J Physiol Gastrointest Liver Physiol 2009;296:G963–G968.

12. Liu Z, Li N, Neu J. Tight junctions, leaky intestines, and pediatric diseases. Acta Paediatr 2005;94:386–93.

13. Alterations of the intestinal barrier in patients with autism spectrum disorders and in their first-degree relatives. J Pediatr Gastroenterol Nutr 2010;51:418–24.

14. Bresnanhan M, Hornig M, Schultz AF, et al. Association of maternal report of infant and toddler gastrointestinal symptoms with autism: evidence from a prospective birth cohort. JAMA Psychiatry 2015;72:466–74.

15. Stoltenberg C, Schjolberg S, Bresnahan M, et al. The Autism Birth Cohort (ABC): a paradigm for gene-environment-timing research. Mol Psychiatry 2010;15:676–80.

16. Sandin S, Hultman CM, Kolevzon A, et al. Advancing maternal age is associated with increasing risk for autism: a review and meta-analysis. J Am Acad Child Adolesc Psychiatry 2012;51:477–86.

17. Durkin MS, Maenner MJ, Newschaffer CJ, et al. Advanced paternal age and the risk of autism spectrum disorder. Am J Epidemiol 2008;168:1268–76.

18. Maimburg RD, Vaeth M. Perinatal risk factors and infantile autism. Acta Psychiatr Scand 2006;114:257–64.

19. Glasson EJ, Bower C, Petterson B, et al. Perinatal factors and the development of autism. A population study. Arch Gen Psychiatry 2004;61:618–27.

20. Ornoy A, Weinstein-Fudim L, Ergaz Z. Prenatal factors associated with autism spectrum disorder (ASD). Reproductive Toxicology 2015;56:155–69.

21. American Psychiatric Association. Diagnostic and statistical manual of mental disorders. Fifth edition. Arlington, VA: American Psychiatric Association, 2013.

22. Gillgerg C, Wing L. Autism: not an extremely rare disorder. Acta Psychiatr Scand 1999;99:399–406.

23. Blumberg SJ, Bramlett MD, Kogan MD, et al. Changes in prevalence of parent-reported autism spectrum disorder in school-age U.S. children: 2007 to 2011–2012. Natl Health Stat Rep 2013;65:1–11.

24. Wakefield AJ, Anthony A, Schepelmann S, et al. Persistent measles virus infection and immunodeficiency in children with autism, ileo-colonic lymphoid nodular hyperplasia and non-specific colitis. Gut 1998;42(Suppl 1):A86.

25. Wakefield AJ, Montgomery SM. Autism, viral infection and measles-mumps-rubella vaccination. IMAJ 1999;1:183–87.

26. Hornig M, Briese T, Buie T, et al. Lack of association between measles virus vaccine and autism with enteropathy: a case control study. PLoS One 2008;3(9):e3140.

27. Chez MG, Guido-Estrada N. Immune therapy in autism: historical experience and future directions with immunomodulatory therapy. Neurotherapeutics 2010;7:293–301.

28. Bouboulis DA, Mast PA. Infection-induced autoimmune encephalopathy: Treatment with intravenous immune globulin therapy. A report of six patients. Int J Neurology Res 2016;2:256–58.

29. Lieneman CC, Brabson LA, Highlander A, et al. Parent–child interaction therapy: current perspectives. Psychol Res Behav Manage 2017;10:239–56.

30. Zlomke KR, Jeter K. Comparative effectiveness of parent-child interaction therapy for children with and without autism spectrum disorder. J Autism Dev Disord 2019 Mar 12. doi: 10.1007/s10803-019-03960-y. [Epub ahead of print].

31. Zimmer-Gembeck MJ, Kerin JL, Webb HJ, et al. Improved perceptions of emotion regulation and reflective functioning in parents: two additional positive outcomes of parent-child interaction therapy. Behav Ther 2019;50(2):340–52.

32. Acosta J, Garcia D, Bagner DM. Parent-child interaction therapy for children with developmental delay: the role of sleep problems. J Dev Behav Pediatr 2019;40(3):183–91.

33. Younger DS. PANDAS plus autism: treatment with IVIg (editorial). Int J Neurol Res 2016;2:224–25.

34. Jyonouchi H, Geng L, Streck DL, et al. Immunological characterization and transcription profiling of peripheral blood (PB) monocytes in children with autism spectrum disorders (ASD) and specific polysaccharide antibody deficiency (SPAD): case study. J Neuroinflammation 2012;9:4.

35. Saxena S, Rauch SL. Functional neuroimaging and the neuroanatomy of obsessive-compulsive disorder. Psychiatr Clin North Am 2000;23(3):563–86.

36. Ting JT, Feng G. Glutamatergic synaptic dysfunction and obsessive-compulsive disorder. Curr Chem Genomics 2008;2:62–75.

37. Shin DJ, Jung WH, He Y, et al. The effects of pharmacological treatment on functional brain connectome in obsessive-compulsive disorder. Biol Psychiatry 2014;75(8):606–14.

38. Teixeira AL, Rodrigues DH, Marques AH, et al. Searching for the immune basis of obsessive-compulsive disorder. Neuroimmunomodulation 2014;21(2-3):152–58.

39. Cubo E, Gabriel y Galan JM, et al. Prevalence of tics in schoolchildren in central Spain: a population-based study. Pediatric Neurology 2011;45:100–08.

40. Bloch MH, Leckman JF. Clinical course of Tourette syndrome. Journal of Psychosomatic Research 2009;67:497–501.

41. Jalenques I, Galland F, Malet L, et al. Quality of life in adults with Gilles de la Tourette Syndrome. BMC Psychiatry 2012;12:109.

42. Scahill L, Erenberg G, Berlin CM, J, et al. Contemporary assessment and pharmacotherapy of Tourette syndrome. NeuroRx: The Journal of the American Society for Experimental NeuroTherapeutics 2006;3:192–206.

43. Woods DW, Piacentini J, Chang SW, et al. Managing Tourette Syndrome: A Behavioral Intervention for Children and Adolescents. New York: Oxford University Press, 2008.

44. Peterson AL. Psychosocial management of tics and intentional repetitive behaviors associated with Tourette syndrome. In: Woods DW, Piacentini J, Walkup JT, editors. Treating Tourette Syndrome and Tic Disorders: A Guide for Practitioners. New York: Guilford Press, 2007; 154–84.

CHAPTER 11: SORE THROATS LEAD TO SORE HEADS: ON THE LOOKOUT FOR PANDAS AND PANS

1. Younger DS, Bouboulis DA. Immune pathogenesis pediatric autoimmune neuropsychiatric disorders associated with group A β-hemolytic streptococcal infections (PANDAS). Int J Neurol Res 2015;1:5–7.

2. Budman CL, Kerjakovic M, Bruun RD. Viral infection and tic exacerbation. J Am Acad Child Adolesc Psychiatry 1997;36:162.

3. Ercan TE, Ercan G, Severge B, Arpaozu M, Karasu G. Mycoplasma pneumoniae infection and obsessive-compulsive disease: a case report. J Child Neurol 2008;23:338–40.

4. Riedel M, Straube A, Schwarz MJ, Wilske B, Muller N. Lyme disease presenting as Tourette's syndrome. Lancet 1998;351:418–19.

5. Pavone P, Bianchini R, Parano E, et al. Anti-brain antibodies in PANDAS versus uncomplicated streptococcal infection. Pediatr Neurol 2004;30(2):107–10.

6. Murphy TK, Storch EA, Lewin EA, Edge PJ, Goodman WK. Clinical factors associated with PANDAS. J Pediatr 2012;160:314–19.

7. Murphy TK, Sajid M, Soto O, Shapira N, Edge P, Yang M, Lewis MH, Goodman WK. Detecting pediatric autoimmune neuropsychiatric disorders associated with streptococcus in children with obsessive-compulsive disorder and tics. Biol Psychiatry 2004;55:61–68.

8. Moleculera. PANS and PANDAS diagnosis and treatment. 2016; http://www.moleculeralabs.com/pandas-pans-diagnosis-and-treatment/.

9. Cox CJ, Sharma M, Leckman JF, Zuccolo J, Zuccolo A, Kovoor A, et al. Brain human monoclonal autoantibody from sydenham chorea targets dopaminergic neurons in transgenic mice and signals dopamine d2 receptor: implications in human disease. J Immunol 2013;191:5524–41.

10. Kirvan CA, Swedo SE, Heuser JS, Cunningham MW. Mimicry and autoantibody-mediated neuronal cell signaling in sydenham chorea. Nat Med 2003;9:914–20.

11. Younger DS, Mast PA, Bouboulis DA. Baseline immunoglobulin levels predict achievement of remission at one year following IVIg therapy. J Neurol Neurosurg 2016;3(3):125.

12. Allen AJ, Leonard HL, Swedo SE. Case study: a new infection-triggered autoimmune subtype of pediatric OCD and Tourette's syndrome. J Am Acad Child Adolesc Psychiatry 1995;34:307–11.

13. Hersh ALB, Geng A, Cushing-Ruby H, et al. Resolution of PANDAS like symptoms by IVIg in a patient with specific antibody deficiency against polysaccharide antigens (Abstract). J Allergy Clin Immunol 2006;117:S519.

14. Younger DS. Pediatric Autoimmune Neuropsychiatric Disorders Associated with Group A Streptococcal Infection and the Impact of Intravenous of Intravenous Immune Globulin Treatment. Master's Essay in Epidemiology, Columbia University, Mailman School of Public Health, May 2016.

15. Younger DS, Mast PA, Bouboulis DA. PANDAS: baseline immunoglobulin levels predict achievement of remission at one year following IVIg therapy. J Neurol Neurosurg 2016;3(2):122.

16. Younger DS, Chen X. IVIg therapy in PANDAS: analysis of the current literature. J Neurol Neurosurg 2016;3(3):125.

17. Younger DS. Autoimmune encephalitides. World Journal of Neuroscience 2017;7:327–61.

CHAPTER 12: THE GUT-BRAIN CONNECTION: CELIAC DISEASE AND BEYOND

1. O'Bryan T. You Can Fix Your Brain. New York: Rodale Books, 2018.

2. Round JL, Mazmanian SK. The gut microbiota shapes intestinal immune responses during health and disease. Nature Reviews: Immunology 2009;9(5):313–23.

3. Kelly JR, Kennedy PJ, Cryan JF, et al. Breaking down the barriers: the gut microbiome, intestinal permeability and stress-related psychiatric disorders. Front Cell Neurosci 2015;9:392.

4. Currie S, Hadjivassiliou M, Clark MJR, et al. Should we be "nervous" about coeliac disease? Brain abnormalities in patients with coeliac disease referred for neurological opinion. J Neurol Neurosurg Psychiatry 2012;83:1216–21.

5. Gabrielli M, Cremonini F, Fiore G, et al. Association between migraine and Celiac disease: Results from a preliminary case-control and therapeutic study. Am J Gastroenterol 2003;98:625–29.

6. Ludvigsson JF, Sellgren C, Runeson B, et al. Increased suicide risk in coeliac disease—a Swedish nationwide cohort study. Dig Liver Dis 2011;43(8):616–22.

7. Ludvigsson JF, Reichenberg A, Hultman CM, et al. A nationwide study of the association between Celiac disease and the risk of autistic spectrum disorders. JAMA Psychiatry 2013;70(11):1224–30.

8. Sekirov I, Russell S.L, Antunes L.C, et al. Gut microbiota in health and disease. Physiol Rev 2010;90:859–904.

9. Furness JB. The enteric nervous system and neurogastroenterology. Nat Rev Gastroenterol Hepatol 2012;9:286–94.

10. Hadjivassiliou M, Grünewald RA, Lawden M, et al. Headache and CNS white matter abnormalities associated with gluten sensitivity. Neurology 2001;56:385–88.

11. Faulkner-Hogg KB, Selby WS, Loblay RH. Dietary analysis in symptomatic patients with coeliac disease on a gluten-free diet: the role of trace amounts of gluten and non-gluten food intolerances. Scand J Gastroenterol 1999;34:784–89.

12. Saito E, Doi H, Kurihara K, et al. The validation of the Wheat Gluten ELISA Kit. J AOAC Int 2019 Feb 26. doi: 10.5740/jaoacint.19-0005. [Epub ahead of print].

13. Zhang J, Portela SB, Horrell JB, et al. An integrated, accurate, rapid, and economical handheld consumer gluten detector. Food Chemistry 2019;275:446–56.

14. Connan V, Marcon MA, Mahmud FH. Online education for gluten-free diet teaching: Development and usability testing of an e-learning module for children with concurrent Celiac disease and type 1 diabetes. Pediatr Diabetes 2019 Jan 16. doi: 10.1111/pedi.12815. [Epub ahead of print].

15. Parzanese I, Qehajaj D, Patrinicola F, et al. Celiac disease: from pathophysiology to treatment. World J Gastrointest Pathophysiol 2017;8(2):27–38.

16. Sansotta N, Amirikian K, Guandalini S, Jericho H. Celiac Disease Symptom Resolution: Effectiveness of the Gluten-free Diet. J. Pediatr. Gastroenterol. Nutr. 2018;66:48–52.

17. Molina-Torres G, Rodriguez-Arrastia M, Roman P, et al. Stress and the gut microbiota-brain axis. Behav Pharmacol 2019 Mar 5. [Epub ahead of print].

18. Flowers SA, Ellingrod VL. The microbiome in mental health: potential contribution of gut microbiota in disease and pharmacotherapy management. Pharmacotherapy 2015;35(10):910–16.

19. Smythies LE, Smythies JR. Microbiota, the immune system, black moods and the brain-melancholia updated. Frontiers in Human Neuroscience 2014;8:720.

CHAPTER 13: CONCUSSIONS LEAVE THEIR MARK

1. Barlow KM, Crawford S, Stevenson A, et al. Epidemiology of postconcussion syndrome in pediatric mild traumatic brain injury. Pediatrics 2010;126:e374–e381.

2. Vargas G, Rabinowitz A, Meyer J, et al. Predictors and prevalence of postconcussion depression symptoms in collegiate athletes. Journal of Athletic Training 2015;50:250–55.

3. Ilie G, Boak A, Adlaf EM, et al. Prevalence and correlates of traumatic brain injuries among adolescents. JAMA 2013;309:2550–52.

4. Younger DS. Hashimoto encephalopathy: impact of concussion. World Journal of Neuroscience 2018;8:108–12.

5. Mondello S, Muller U, Jeromin A, Streeter J, Hayes RL, Wang KK. Blood-based diagnostics of traumatic brain injuries. Expert Rev Mol Diagn 2011;11(1):65–78.

6. Tagge CA, Fisher AM, Minaeva OV, et al. Concussion, microvascular injury, and early tauopathy in young athletes after impact head injury and an impact concussion mouse model. Brain 2018;141:422–58.

7. Barlow KM, Crawford S, Stevenson A, et al. Epidemiology of postconcussion syndrome in pediatric mild traumatic brain injury. Pediatrics 2010;126:e374–e381.

8. Stern RA, Riley DO, Daneshvar DH, et al. Long-term consequences of repetitive brain trauma: chronic traumatic encephalopathy. PM&R 2011;3 (10 suppl 2):S460–S467.

9. Richard YF, Swaine BR, Sylvestre MP, Lesage A, Zhang X, Feldman DE. The association between traumatic brain injury and suicide: are kids at risk? Am J Epidemiol 2015;182(2):177–84.

10. https://www.fda.gov/newsevents/newsroom/pressannouncements/ucm596531
.htm.

11. McKee AC, Stein TD, Kiernan PT, Alvarez VE. The neuropathology of chronic traumatic encephalopathy. Brain Pathology (Zurich, Switzerland) 2015; 25:350–64.

12. Younger DS. Autoimmune encephalitides. World Journal of Neuroscience 2017;7:327–61.

13. Younger DS. Serial Brain Positron Emission Tomography Fused to Magnetic Resonance Imaging in Post-Infectious and Autoantibody-Associated Autoimmune Encephalitis. World Journal of Neuroscience 2019; 9:153–156.

14. Coughlin JM, Yang T, Rebman AW, Kortte KB, Du Y, Mathews WB et al. (2018) Imaging Glial Activation in Patients with Post-Treatment Lyme Disease Symptoms: A Pilot Study Using [11C]DPA-713 PET. Journal of Neuroinflammation, 15, 346.

15. Younger DS. Hashimoto Encephalopathy: Impact of Concussion. World Journal of Neuroscience 2018; 8:108–112.

16. Burns DD. Feeling Good: The New Mood Therapy. New York: HarperCollins, 2000.

17. Scogin F, Jamison C, Gochneaut K. The comparative efficacy of cognitive and behavioral bibliotherapy for mildly and moderately depressed older adults. J Consul Clin Psychol 1989;57:403–07.

18. Brooker SM, Gobeske KT, Chen J, et al. Hippocampal bone morphogenetic protein signaling mediates behavioral effects of antidepressant treatment. Mol Psychiatry 2017;22:910–19.

CHAPTER 14: NEUROENDOCRINE AND MAST CELL ACTIVITY DETERMINE HOW YOU RESPOND TO STRESS

1. Justice NJ. The relationship between stress and Alzheimer's disease. Neurobiol Stress 2018;8:127–33.

2. Kempuraj D, Selvakumar GP, Thangavel R, et al. Mast cell activation in brain injury, stress, and post-traumatic stress disorder and Alzheimer's disease pathogenesis. Front Neurosci 2017;11:703.

3. Lurie DI. An integrative approach to neuroinflammation in psychiatric disorders and neuropathic pain. J Exp Neurosci 2018;12:1179069518793639.

4. Theoharides TC, Alysandratos KD, Angelidou A, et al. Mast cells and inflammation. Biochim Biophys Acta 2012;1822:21–33.

5. Kempuraj D, Thangavel R, Selvakumar GP, et al. Brain and peripheral atypical inflammatory mediators potentiate neuroinflammation and neurodegeneration. Front Cell Neurosci 2017;11:216.

6. Gupta K, Harvima IT. Mast cell-neural interactions contribute to pain and itch. Immunol Rev 2018;282:168–87.

7. Theoharides TC, Kavalioti M. Stress, inflammation and natural treatments. J Biol Regul Homeost Agents 2018;32:1345–47.

8. Holzer P, Farzi A, Hassan AM, et al. Visceral inflammation and immune activation stress the brain. Front Immunol 2017;8:1613.

9. Esposito P, Gheorghe D, Kandere K, et al. Acute stress increases permeability of the blood-brain-barrier through activation of brain mast cells. Brain Res 2001;888:117–27.

10. Karagkouni A, Alevizos M, Theoharides TC. Effect of stress on brain inflammation and multiple sclerosis. Autoimmun Rev 2013;12:947–53.

11. Norheim KB, Jonsson G, Omdal R. Biological mechanisms of chronic fatigue. Rheumatology (Oxford) 2011;50:1009–18.

12. Afrin LB, Self S, Menk J, et al. Characterization of mast cell activation syndrome. Am J Med Sci 2016;353(3):207–15.

13. Younger DS. Hashimoto's thyroiditis and encephalopathy. World Journal of Neuroscience 2017;7:307–26.

14. Brain L, Jellinek EH, Ball K. Hashimoto's disease and encephalopathy. Lancet 1966;288:512–14.

15. Jellinek EH, Ball K. Hashimoto's disease, encephalopathy, and splenic atrophy. Lancet 1976;307:1248.

16. Graus F, Titulaer MJ, Balu R, et al. A clinical approach to diagnosis of autoimmune encephalitis. Lancet Neurology 2016;15:391–404.

17. Bien CG, Vincent A, Barnett MH, et al. Immunopathology of autoantibody-associated encephalitides: clues for pathogenesis. Brain 2012;135:1622–38.

18. Tagge CA, Fisher AM, Minaeva OV, et al. Concussion, microvascular injury, and early tauopathy in young athletes after impact head injury and an impact concussion mouse model. Brain 2018;141:422–58.

CHAPTER 15: PORPHYRIA: A MISDIAGNOSED NEUROGENETIC DISORDER

1. González-Arriaza HL, Bostwick JM. Acute porphyrias: a case report and review. Am J Psychiatry. 2003;160(3):450–459

2. Crimlisk HL. The little imitator—porphyria: a neuropsychiatric disorder. J Neurol Neurosurg Psychiatry. 1997;62(4):319–328.

3. Puy H, Deybach JC, Lamoril J, et al. Molecular epidemiology and diagnosis of PBG deaminase gene defects in acute intermittent porphyria. Am J Hum Genet 1997;60:1373–1383.

4. Puy H, Gouya L, Deybach JC. Porphyrias. Lancet 2010; 375:924–37.

5. Zhang Q, Raoof M, Chen Y, et al. Circulating mitochondrial DAMPs cause inflammatory responses to injury. Nature. 2010;464(7285):104–107.

6. Frimat M, Tabarin F, Dimitrov JD et al Complement activation by heme as a secondary hit for atypical hemolytic uremic syndrome. Blood 2013; 122:282–92.

7. Storjord E, Dahl JA, Landsem A, et al. Systemic inflammation in acute intermittent porphyria: a case-control study. Clin Exp Immunol. 2016;187(3):466–479.

8. Tracy JA, Dyck PJ. Porphyria and its neurologic manifestations In: Biller J, Ferro JM, editors. Handbook of clinical neurology. Amsterdam: Elsevier, 2014:839–49.

9. Younger DS, Tanji K. Demyelinating neuropathy in genetically confirmed acute intermittent porphyria. Muscle Nerve 2015; 52:916–917.

CHAPTER 16: CHRONIC FATIGUE SYNDROME: RELIEF FOR EXHAUSTED PATIENTS

1. Davies S, Crawley E. Chronic fatigue syndrome in children aged 11 years old and younger. Arch Dis Child 2008;93:419–22.

2. Crawley EM, Edmond AM, Sterne JAC. Unidentified chronic fatigue syndrome/myalgic encephalomyelitis (CFS/ME) is a major cause of school absence: surveillance outcomes from school-based clinics. BMJ Open 2011;1(2):e000252.

3. Ramsay AM. Postviral Fatigue Syndrome. The Saga of Royal Free Disease. London: Gower, 1986.

4. Ramsay AM. Myalgic Encephalomyelitis and Postviral Fatigue States. Second edition. London: Gower, 1988.

5. Ortega-Hernandez OD, Shoenfeld Y. Infection, vaccination, and autoantibodies in chronic fatigue syndrome, cause or coincidence? Ann N Y Acad Sci 2009;1173: 600–09.

6. Ablashi DV, Eastman HB, Owen CB, et al. Frequent HHV-6 reactivation in multiple sclerosis (MS) and chronic fatigue syndrome (CFS) patients. J Clin Virol 2000;16:179–91.

7. Morris G, Berk M, Galecki P, et al. The emerging role of autoimmunity in myalgic encephalomyelitis/chronic fatigue syndrome (ME/CFS). Mol Neurobiol 2014;49(2):741–56.

8. Sotzny F, Blanco J, Capelli E, et al. Myalgic encephalomyelitis/chronic fatigue syndrome—evidence for an autoimmune disease. Autoimmun Rev 2018;17:601–09.

9. Calabrese LH, Davis ME, Wilke WS. Chronic fatigue syndrome and a disorder resembling Sjorgen's syndrome: preliminary report. Clin Infect Dis 1994;18(suppl 1): S28–S31.

10. Gherardi R, Authier F. Macrophagic myofasciitis: characterization and pathophysiology. Lupus 2012;21:184–89.

11. Katz BZ, Shiraishi Y, Mears CJ, et al. Chronic fatigue syndrome following infectious mononucleosis in adolescents. Pediatrics 2009;124(1):189–93.

12. Hatcher S1, House A. Life events, difficulties and dilemmas in the onset of chronic fatigue syndrome: a case-control study. Psychol Med 2003;33(7):1185–92.

13. Lloyd A, Hickie I, Wakefield D, et al. A double-blind, placebo-controlled trial of intravenous immunoglobulin therapy in patients with chronic fatigue syndrome. Am J Med 1990;89:561–68.

14. Tomijenovic L, Colafrancesco S, Perrricone C, et al. Postural orthostatic tachycardia with chronic fatigue after HPV vaccination as part of the "autoimmune/auto-inflammatory syndrome induced by adjuvants": case report and literature review. Journal of Investigative Medicine High Impact Case Reports 2014;2(1):2324709614527812.

CHAPTER 17: LYME DISEASE: THE GREAT IMITATOR OR THE GREAT TRIGGER?

1. Bai Y, Narayan K, Dail D, Sondey M, Hodzic E, Barthold SW, Pachner AR, Cadavid D. Spinal cord involvement in the nonhuman primate model of Lyme disease. Lab Invest 2004;84(2):160–72.

2. Ramesh G, Didier PJ, England JD, et al. Inflammation in the pathogenesis of Lyme neuroborreliosis. Am J Pathol 2015;185(5):1344–60.

3. Centers for Disease Control and Prevention. MMWR Mort Morb Wkly Rep 2014;61:1–125.

4. Garin C, Bujadoux A. Paralysis by ticks. 1922. Clin Infect Dis 1992;16:168–69.

5. Bannwarth A. Chronische lymphozytare meningitis, entzundliche polyneuritis und "Rheumatismus." Arch Psychiat Nervenkr 1941;113:284–376.

6. Sköldenberg B, Stiernstedt G, Gårde A, et al. Chronic meningitis caused by a penicillin-sensitive microorganism? Lancet 1983;2:75–78.

7. Steere AC, Malawista SE, Hardin JA, et al. Erythema chronicum migrans and Lyme arthritis. The enlarging spectrum. Ann Intern Med 1977;86:685–98.

8. Steere AC, Malawista SE, Snydman DR, et al. Lyme arthritis: an epidemic of oligoarticular arthritis in children and adults in three Connecticut communities. Arthritis Rheum 1977;20:7–17.

9. Reik L, Steere AC, Bartenhagen NH, et al. Neurological abnormalities of Lyme disease. Medicine 1979;58:281–94.

10. Pachner AR, Steere AC. The triad of neurological manifestations of Lyme disease: meningitis, cranial neuritis, and radiculoneuritis. Neurology 1985;35:47–53.

11. Halperin JJ, Little BW, Coyle PK, et al. Lyme disease: cause of a treatable neuropathy. Neurology 1987;37:1700–06.

12. Halperin JJ, Luft BJ, Anand AK, et al. Lyme neuroborreliosis: central nervous system manifestations. Neurology 1989;39:753–59.

13. Steere AC. Lyme disease. N Engl J Med 1989;321:586–96.

14. Ackermann R, Rehse-Küpper B, Gollmer E, et al. Chronic neurologic manifestations of erythema migrans borreliosis. Ann NY Acad Sci 1988;539:16–23.

15. Pachner AR, Duray P, Steere AC. Central nervous system manifestations of Lyme disease. Arch Neurol 1989;46:790–95.

16. Logigian EL, Kaplan RF, Steere AC. Chronic neurologic manifestations of Lyme disease. N Engl J Med 1990;323:1438–44.

17. Younger DS, Wu WE, Hardy C, Perry N, Gonen O. Lyme neuroborreliosis and proton MR spectroscopy: preliminary results from an urban referral

center employing strict CDC criteria for case selection. Neurology 2012;78(Suppl1):PO3.246.

18. Logigian EL, Johnson KA, Kijewski MF, et al. Reversible cerebral hypoperfusion in Lyme encephalopathy. Neurology 1997;49:1661–70.

19. Hansen K. Lyme neuroborreliosis: improvements of the laboratory diagnosis and a survey of epidemiological and clinical features in Denmark 1985-1990. Acta Neurol Scand 1994;151(Suppl):1–44.

20. Sindern E, Malin JP. Phenotypic analysis of cerebrospinal fluid over the course of Lyme meningoradiculitis. Acta Cytol 1995;39:73–75.

21. Horowitz RI. Why Can't I Get Better? Solving the Mystery of Lyme & Chronic Disease. New York: St. Martin Press, 2013;
    Horowitz RI. How Can I Get Better? An Action Plan for Treating Resistant Lyme & Chronic Disease. New York: St. Martin's Griffin, 2017.

22. Adapted from http://www.cangetbetter.com/medical-center.

23. https://www.aan.com/guidelines/home/getguidelinecontent/241.

24. Adapted from https://www.aan.com/Guidelines/home/GetGuidelineContent/241.

CHAPTER 18: SPONDYLOARTHROPATHY: I-CUBED AND GENETICALLY PREDETERMINED JOINT DISEASES

1. Manasson J, Shen N, Garcia Ferrer HR, et al. Gut microbiota perturbations in reactive arthritis and postinfectious spondyloarthritis. Arthritis Rheumatol 2018;70(2):242–54.

2. Lee YC, Nassikas NJ, Clauw DJ. The role of the central nervous system in the generation and maintenance of chronic pain in rheumatoid arthritis, osteoarthritis and fibromyalgia. Arthritis Res Ther 2011;13:211.

3. Sluka KA, Berkley KJ, O'Connor MI, et al. Neural and psychosocial contributions to sex differences in knee osteoarthritic pain. Biol Sex Differ 2012;3:26.

4. Pathnan EM, Inman RD. Pain in spondyloarthritis: a neuro-immune reaction. Best Pract Clin Rheumatol 2017;31(6):830–84.

5. Ikeuchi M, Izumi M, Aso K, et al. Clinical characteristics of pain originating from intra-articular structures of the knee joint in patients with medial knee osteoarthritis. Springerplus 2013;2:628.

6. Wu Q, Inman RD, Davis KD. Neuropathic pain in ankylosing spondylitis: a psychophysics and brain imaging study. Arthritis Rheum 2013;65:1494–503.

7. Low LA, Millecamps M, Seminowicz DA, et al. Nerve injury causes long-term attentional deficits in rats. Neurosci Lett 2012;529:103–07.

8. Manasson J, Scher JU. Spondyloarthritis and the microbiome: new insights from an ancient hypothesis. Curr Rheumatol Rep 2015;17(2):10.

9. Siala M, Gdoura R, Fourati H, et al. Broad-range PCR, cloning and sequencing of the full 16S rRNA gene for detection of bacterial DNA in synovial fluid samples of Tunisian patients with reactive and undifferentiated arthritis. Arthritis Res Ther 2009;11(4):R102.

10. Brewerton DA, Caffrey M, Nicholls A, Walters D, Oates JK, James DC. Reiter's disease and HL-A 27. Lancet 1973;302(7836):996–98.

11. Bowness P, Ridley A, Shaw J, et al. Th17 cells expressing KIR3DL2+ and responsive to HLA-B27 homodimers are increased in ankylosing spondylitis. J Immunol 2011;186:2672–80.

12. Sieper J, Rudwaleit M, Braun J, et al. Diagnosing reactive arthritis: role of clinical setting in the value of serologic and microbiologic assays. Arthritis Rheum 2002;46(2):319–27.

13. Hammer RE, Maila SD, Richardson JA, et al. Spontaneous inflammatory disease in transgenic rates expressing HLA-B27 and human beta 2m: an animal model of HLA-B27-associated human disorders. Cell 199063:1099–112.

14. Rath HC, Herfarth HH, Ikeda JS, et al. Normal luminal bacteria, especially Bacteriodes species, mediated chronic colitis, gastritis, and arthritis in HLA-B27/human beta2 microglobulin transgenic rats. J Clin Invest 1996;98:945–53.

15. Glatigny S, Fert I, Blaton MA, et al. Proinflammatory Th17 cells are expanded and induced by dendritic cells in spondyloarthritis-prone HLA-B27-transgenic rats. Arthritis Rheum 2012;64:110–20.

16. DeLay ML, Turner MJ, Klenk EI, et al. HLA-B27 misfolding and the unfolded protein response augment interleukin-23 production and are associated with Th17 activation in transgenic rats. Arthritis Rheum 2009;60:2633–43.

17. Scher JU, Littman DR, Abramson SB. Microbiome in inflammatory arthritis and human rheumatic diseases. Arthritis Rheum 2016;68(1):35–45.

18. National Ankylosing Spondylitis Society. Looking ahead: best practice for the care of people with ankylosing spondylitis. http://nass.co.uk/campaigning/looking-ahead/.

19. Song IH, Poddubnyy DA, Rudwaleit M, et al. Benefits and risks of ankylosing spondylitis treatment with nonsteroidal antiinflammatory drugs. Arthritis Rheum 2008;58:929–38.

20. Sieper J, Lenaerts J, Wollenhaupt J. et al. Efficacy and safety of infliximab plus naproxen versus naproxen alone in patients with early, active axial spondyloarthritis: results from the double-blind, placebo-controlled INFAST study, part 1. Ann Rheum Dis 2014;73:101–07.

21. van der Heijde D, Kivitz A, Schiff MH. et al. Efficacy and safety of adalimumab in patients with ankylosing spondylitis: results of a multicenter, randomized, double-blind, placebo-controlled trial. Arthritis Rheum 2006;54:2136–46.

22. Pinto Carneiro JB, Pinto de Souza T, Antunes de Oliveira TML, et al. Coexistence of spondyloarthritis and joint hypermobility syndrome: rare or unknown association? Reumatismo 2017;69(3):126–30.

23. Rodgers KR, Gui J, Dinulos MB, et al. Ehlers-Danlos syndrome hypermobility type is associated with rheumatic diseases. Sci Rep 2017;7:39636.

CHAPTER 19: AUTOIMMUNE ENCEPHALITIS: A BRAIN ON FIRE

1. Goldsmith CA, Rogers DP. The case for autoimmunity in the etiology of schizophrenia. Pharmacotherapy 2008;28:730–41.

2. Ching KH, Burbelo PD, Carlson PJ, et al. High levels of anti-GAD65 and anti-Ro52 autoantibodies in a patient with major depressive disorder showing psychomotor disturbance. J Neuroimmunol 2010;222:87–89.

3. Cahalan S. Brain on Fire: My Month of Madness. New York, Free Press, 2012.

4. Dalmau J, Tüzün E, Wu HY, et al. Paraneoplastic anti-N-methyl-D-aspartate receptor encephalitis associated with ovarian teratoma. Ann Neurol 2007;61(1):25–36.

5. Sansing LH, Tüzin E, Ko MW, et al. A patient with encephalitis associated with NMDA receptor antibodies. Nat Clin Pract Neurol 2007; 3:291–296.

6. Bien CG, Vincent A, Barnett MH, et al. Immunopathology of autoantibody-associated encephalitides: clues for pathogenesis. Brain 2012;135:1622–38.

7. Park DC, Reuter-Lorenz P. The adaptive brain: aging and neurocognitive scaffolding. Annual Rev Psychol 2009;60:173–96.

8. Bennett DLH, Vincent A. Autoimmune pain. Neurology 2012;79:1080–81.

9. Lahoria R, Pittock SJ, Gadoth A, et al. Clinical-pathologic correlations in voltage-gated Kv1 potassium channel complex-subtyped autoimmune painful polyneuropath. Muscle Nerve 2017;55(4):520–25.

10. Klein CJ, Lennon VA, Aston PA, et al. Chronic pain as a manifestation of potassium channel-complex autoimmunity. Neurology 2012;79:1136–44.

11. Ohkawa T, Fukata Y, Yamasaki M, et al. Autoantibodies to epilepsy-related LGI1 in limbic encephalitis neutralize LGI1-ADAM22 interaction and reduce synaptic AMPA receptor. Journal of Neuroscience 2013;33:18161–74.

12. Younger D. Limbic encephalitis associated with voltage-gated potassium channel-complex antibodies: Patient report and literature review. World Journal of Neuroscience 2017:7:19–31.

CHAPTER 20: ALZHEIMER'S DISEASE AND OTHER DEMENTIAS: AUTOIMMUNE INSIGHTS

1. Nelson PT, Alafuzoff I, Bigio EH, et al. Correlation of Alzheimer's disease neuropathologic changes with cognitive status: a review of the literature. J Neuropath Exp Neurol 2012;71:362–81.

2. Readhead B, Haure-Mirande JV, Funk CC, et al. Multiscale analysis of independent Alzheimer's cohorts finds disruption of molecular, genetic, and clinical networks by human herpesvirus. Neuron 2018;99:64–82.

3. Aisen PS, Cummings J, Jack CR, et al. On the path to 2025: understanding the Alzheimer's disease continuum. Alzheimers Res Ther 2017;9(1):60.

4. Wagner M, Wolf S, Reischies FM, et al. Biomarker validation of a cued recall memory deficit in prodromal Alzheimer disease. Neurology 2012;78:379–86.

5. Ubhi K, Masliah E. Alzheimer's disease: recent advances and future perspectives. J Alzheimers Dis 2013;33:S185–S194.

6. Jekel K, Damian M, Wattmo C, et al. Mild cognitive impairment and deficits in instrumental activities of daily living: a systematic review. Alzheimers Res Ther 2015;7:17.

7. Loeffler DA. Intravenous immunoglobulin and Alzheimer's disease: what now? J Neuroinflammation 2013;10:70.

8. Jankovic J. Parkinson's disease: clinical features and diagnosis. J Neurol Neurosurg Psychiatry 2008;79:368–76.

9. Wakabayashi K, Takahashi H, Takeda S, et al. Parkinson's disease: the presence of Lewy bodies in Auerbach's and Meissner's plexuses. Acta Neuropathol (Berl) 1988;76:217–21.

10. Bertram L, Tanzi RE. The genetics of Alzheimer's disease. Prog Mol Biol Transl Sci 2012;107:79–100.

11. Jensen-Dahm C, Waldemar G, Staehelin Jensen T, et al. Autonomic dysfunction in patients with mild to moderate Alzheimer's disease. J Alzheimers Dis 2015;47(3):681–89.

12. Lyons MK, Caselli RJ, Parisi JE. Nonvasculitic autoimmune inflammatory meningoencephalitis as a cause of potentially reversible dementia: report of 4 cases. J Neurosurg 2008;108:1024–27.

13. Wisniewski T, Goni F. Immunotherapy for Alzheimer's disease. Biochem Pharmacol 2014;88:499–507.

14. Wisniewski T, Goni F. Could immunomodulation be used to prevent prion diseases? Expert Rev Anti Infect Ther 2012;10:307–17.

15. Huang Y, Mucke L. Alzheimer mechanisms and therapeutic strategies. Cell 2012;148:1204–22.

16. World Health Organization. International Classification of Functioning, Disability and Health (ICF). Geneva: World Health Organization, 2001.

17. McDermott O, Charlesworth G, Hogervorst E, et al. Psychosocial interventions for people with dementia: a synthesis of systematic reviews. Aging Ment Health 2018;17:1–11.

18. Gitlin LN, Winter L, Vause Earland T, et al. The Tailored Activity Program to reduce behavioral symptoms in individuals with dementia: feasibility, acceptability, and replication potential. Gerontologist 2009;49(3):428–39.

19. Gitlin LN, Winter L, Burke J, et al. Tailored activities to manage neuropsychiatric behaviors in persons with dementia and reduce caregiver burden: a randomized pilot study. Am J Geriatr Psychiatry 2008;16(3):229–39.

20. Flanagan EP, McKeon A, Lennon VA, et al. Autoimmune dementia: clinical course and predictors of immunotherapy response. Mayo Clin Proc 2010;85:881–97.

21. Kelley BJ, Boeve BF, Josephs KA. Young-onset dementia: demographic and etiologic characteristics of 235 patients. Arch Neurol 2008;65:1502–08.

22. Flanagan EP, McKeon A, Lennon VA, et al. Autoimmune dementia: clinical course and predictors of immunotherapy response. Mayo Clin Proc 2010;85:881–97.

23. Knopman DS, Petersen RC. Mild cognitive impairment and mild dementia: a clinical perspective. Mayo Clin Proc 2014;89:1452–59.

24. McKeon A, Marnane M, O'Connell M, et al. Potassium channel antibody associated encephalopathy presenting with a frontotemporal dementia like syndrome. Arch Neurol 2007;64:1528–30.

25. Mateen FJ, Josephs KA, Parisi JE, et al. Steroid-responsive encephalopathy subsequently associated with Alzheimer's disease pathology: a case series. Neurocase 2012;18:1–12.

26. Cutsforth-Gregory JK, McKeon A, Coon EA, et al. Ganglionic antibody level as a predictor of severity of autonomic failure. Mayo Clin Proc 2018;93:1440–47.

27. Younger DS. A postmortem study of a patient with low titer nicotinic acetylcholine receptor ganglionic antibody: Implications for clinical neurologic disease. World Journal of Neuroscience 2019; 9:71-75.

CHAPTER 21: THE SURPRISING LINK BETWEEN COVID-19 AND I-CUBED

1. Zhu N, Zhang D, Wang W, et al. A novel coronavirus from patients with pneumonia in China, 2019. N Engl J Med 2020; 382(8):727–33.

2. Andersen KG, Rambaut A, Lipkin WI, et al. The proximal origin of SARS-CoV-2. Nat Med 2020; 26:450–52.

3. Su S, Wong G, Shi W, et al. Epidemiology, genetic recombination, and pathogenesis of coronaviruses. Trends Microbiol 2016; 24:490–502.

4. Zhong NS, Zheng BJ, Li YM, et al. Epidemiology and cause of severe acute respiratory syndrome (SARS) in Guangdong, People's Republic of China, in February 2003. Lancet 2003; 362:1353–58.

5. Perico L, Benigni A, Casiraghi F, et al. Immunity, endothelial injury and complement-induced coagulopathy in COVID-19. Nat Rev Nephrol 2021; 17(1):46–64.

6. Mantovani E, Mariotto S, Gabbiani D, et al. Chronic fatigue syndrome: an emerging sequela in COVID-19 survivors? J Neurovirol 2021; 2:1–7.

7. Younger DS. The autoimmune brain: A five-step plan for treating chronic pain, depression, anxiety, fatigue, and attention disorders (book review). IJRMS 2020; 4(12):707–11.

8. Matschke J, Lütgehetmann M, Hagel C, et al. Neuropathology of patients with COVID-19 in Germany: a post-mortem case series. Lancet Neurol 2020; 19(11):919–29.

9. Shi Y, et al. COVID-19 infection: the perspectives on immune responses. Cell Death Differ 2020; 27:1451–54.

10. Xu Z, Shi L, Wang Y, et al. Pathological findings of COVID-19 associated with acute respiratory distress syndrome. Lancet Respir Med 2020; 8:420–22.

11. Puelles VG, Lütgehetmann M, Lindenmeyer MT, et al. Multiorgan and renal tropism of SARS-CoV-2 [published online ahead of print, 2020 May 13]. N Engl J Med 2020; NEJMc2011400.

12. Elliott J, Bodinier B, Whitaker M, et al. COVID-19 mortality in the UK Biobank cohort: revisiting and evaluating risk factors. Eur J Epidemiol 2021; 36(3):299–309.

13. Cheung EW, Zachariah P, Gorelik M, et al. Multisystem inflammatory syndrome related to COVID-19 in previously healthy children and adolescents in New York City. JAMA 2020; 324:294–96.

14. Feldstein LR, Rose EB, Horwitz SM, et al. Multisystem inflammatory syndrome in U.S. children and adolescents. N Engl J Med 2020; 383(4):334–46.

15. Younger DS. Postmortem neuropathology in COVID-19. Brain Pathol. 2021; 31(2):385–86; Younger DS. Coronavirus 2019: clinical and neuropathological aspects. Curr Opin Rheumatol 2021; 33(1):49–57.

16. Younger DS. Postmortem neuropathology in COVID-19. Brain Pathol 2021; 31(2):385–86.

17. Naseri NN, Wang H, Guo J, et al. The complexity of tau in Alzheimer's disease. Neurosci Lett 2019; 705:183–94.

18. Naserkhaki R, Zamanzadeh S, Baharvand H, et al. cis pT231-Tau Drives Neurodegeneration in Bipolar Disorder. ACS Chem Neurosci. 2019; 10(3):1214–21.

19. National Institutes of Health. Post-acute sequelae of SARS-CoV-2 infection initiative: SARS-CoV-2 recovery cohort studies. https://covid19.nih.gov/sites/default/files/2021-02/PASC-ROA-OTA-Recovery-Cohort-Studies.pdf.

20. Davis HE, Assaf GS, McCorkell L, et al. Characterizing long COVID in an international cohort: 7 months of symptoms and their impact. MedRxiv 2020; 20248802.

21. Sudre CH, Murray B, Varsavsky T, et al. Attributes and predictors of Long-COVID: Analysis of COVID cases and their symptoms collected by the Covid Symptoms Study App. medRxiv 2020; 20214494.

22. Cevik M, Tate M, Lloyd O, et al. SARS-CoV-2, SARS-CoV, and MERS-CoV viral load dynamics, duration of viral shedding, and infectiousness: a systematic review and meta-analysis. Lancet Microbe 2021; 2(1):e13–e22.

23. Younger DS. Immunotherapy for the post-infectious sequela of SARS-CoV-2 infection. World J Neurosci 2020; 10:117–20.

24. Mohtadi N, Ghaysouri A, Shirazi S, et al. Recovery of severely ill COVID-19 patients by intravenous immunoglobulin (IVIG) treatment: A case series. Virology 2020; 548:1–5.

25. Ali S, Uddin SM, Shalim E, et al. Hyperimmune anti-COVID-19 IVIG (C-IVIG) treatment in severe and critical COVID-19 patients: A phase I/II randomized control trial. EClinicalMedicine 2021; 36:100926.

26. Harahsheh AS, Dahdah N, Newburger JW, et al. Missed or delayed diagnosis of Kawasaki disease during the 2019 novel coronavirus disease (COVID-19) pandemic. J Pediatr 2020; 222:261–62.

27. Caricchio R, Gallucci M, Dass C., Temple University COVID-19 Research Group, et al. Preliminary predictive criteria for COVID-19 cytokine storm. Ann Rheum Dis 2021; 80(1):88–95.

28. Younger DS. Post-infectious sequela of SARS-COV-2 infection in adults and children: An overview of available agents and clinical responsiveness. Arch Neurol Neurologic Dis 2020; 3:e102.

29. The Autoimmune Brain, https://www.facebook.com/groups/189284839185730.

30. Younger D. Preliminary guidelines for the use of IVIg during COVID-19. World J Neurosci 2021; 11:211–20.

31. McBride L. By now, burnout is a given. The Atlantic. https://www.theatlantic .com/ideas/archive/2021/06/burnout-medical-condition-pandemic/619321/.

32. Lopez Bernal J, Andrews N, Gower C, Gallagher E, et al. Effectiveness of Covid-19 vaccines against the B.1.617.2 (delta) variant. N Engl J Med 2021; 385(7):585–94.

CHAPTER 22: PUTTING IT ALL TOGETHER TO RESOLVE YOUR HEALTH

1. Hohlfeld R. Neurological autoimmune disease and the trimolecular complex of T-lymphocytes. Ann Neurol 1989; 25:531-538.

Index